369 0246917

KU-285-981

A Path to Nursing Excellence

• • • • •

Mary O'Neil Mundinger, DrPH, FAAN, is the Edward M. Kennedy Professor of Health Policy and dean emeritus, Columbia University School of Nursing (CUSON), and former associate dean, Faculty of Medicine, Columbia University. Dean Mundinger led Columbia University School of Nursing for more than 25 years, from a state of near demise to a state of national status as one of the premier schools of nursing in the United States. Dr. Mundinger was instrumental in establishing CUSON's doctor of nurse practioner (DNP) program as a model of advanced clinical practice and its graduates as recognized primary care providers. Dr. Mundinger has been the principal investigator or project director for more than $5 million in funded research. She is the recipient of two *American Journal of Nursing* Book of the Year awards (1981 for *Autonomy in Nursing* and 1984 for *Home Care Controversy: Too Little, Too Late, Too Costly*). Dr. Mundinger has consulted with or has served on the board of directors for multiple health-related corporations, including Welch Allyn, Gentiva, UnitedHealthcare, and Cell Therapeutics. She is the founding president of the Friends of the National Institute for Nursing Research (FNINR), has served as a member of the White House National Steering Committee on Health, and director of the Columbia University World Health Organization Center for International Nursing Development of Advanced Practice, among others. Dr. Mundinger is the recipient of many awards, including the NP of the Year Award (*Nurse Practitioner Journal*); member, the Institute of Medicine; fellow, the New York Academy of Medicine; fellow, American Academy of Nursing; fellow, Robert Wood Johnson Health Policy Program, Institute of Medicine/National Academy of Sciences; and Health Policy staff member, Senator Edward M. Kennedy, Senate Committee on Labor and Human Resources. In addition to her two books, Dr. Mundinger has published widely, including nearly 60 peer-reviewed papers and many invited papers presented to the Institute of Medicine, National Academy of Sciences, National Organization for Nurse Practitioner Faculty, American Association of Colleges of Nursing, American Association of Nurse Practitioners, the Federation of State Medical Boards, the American College Health Association, the American Medical Association, and others.

A Path to Nursing Excellence
The Columbia Experience

•••••

Mary O'Neil Mundinger, DrPH, FAAN

SPRINGER PUBLISHING COMPANY

NEW YORK

Copyright © 2014 Springer Publishing Company, LLC

All rights reserved.

Springer Publishing Company, LLC
11 West 42nd Street
New York, NY 10036
www.springerpub.com

Acquisitions Editor: Margaret Zuccarini
Composition: S4Carlisle Publishing Services

ISBN: 978-0-8261-6952-5
e-book ISBN: 978-0-8261-6953-2

13 14 15 16 17 / 5 4 3 2 1

Library of Congress Cataloging-in-Publication Data
Mundinger, Mary O'Neil, author.
A path to nursing excellence : the Columbia experience / Mary O'Neil Mundinger.
    p. ; cm.
Includes index.
ISBN-13: 978-0-8261-6952-5 — ISBN-10: 0-8261-6952-X — ISBN-13: 978-0-8261-6953-2 (e-book)
I. Title.
[DNLM: 1. Columbia University. School of Nursing. 2. Schools, Nursing—history—Personal Narratives. 3. Education, Nursing—history—Personal Narratives. WY 19]
RT79
610.73071'17471—dc23   2013021405

Special discounts on bulk quantities of our books are available to corporations, professional associations, pharmaceutical companies, health care organizations, and other qualifying groups. If you are interested in a custom book, including chapters from more than one of our titles, we can provide that service as well.
For details, please contact:
Special Sales Department, Springer Publishing Company, LLC
11 West 42nd Street, 15th Floor, New York, NY 10036-8002
Phone: 877-687-7476 or 212-431-4370; Fax: 212-941-7842
E-mail: sales@springerpub.com

Printed in the United States of America by Courier.

• • • • •
───

Dedication

• • • • •

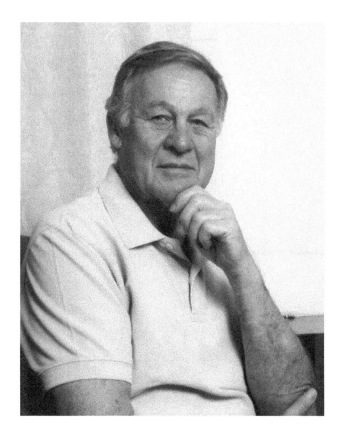

To my beloved husband Paul C. Mundinger

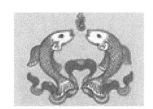

Contents

•••••

• • • • •

Preface

• • • • •

THIS MANUSCRIPT IS A 25-YEAR history of radical change in the nursing profession that emanated from hard-fought innovations at the Columbia University School of Nursing. I was dean from 1985 until 2010, and the cascade of accomplishments of the faculty during my tenure include educational reform, attaining research eminence, building a core of health policy into all of our endeavors and, most profoundly, advancing nursing practice to its most influential and highest levels.

We established independent practice for nurse practitioners for the first time, with full-scope practice including hospital admitting privileges, ER evaluations, and service for a population of 700 underserved patients receiving care at Presbyterian Hospital, one of the nation's premier medical centers. To ensure that our innovation would have broad recognition and strong support, we evaluated the practice in the only randomized controlled trial ever conducted comparing nurse practitioners with physicians in primary care. The results were published as the lead article in the first issue of 2000 in the *Journal of the American Medical Association* (*JAMA*). Our study showed that there were no differences in care, cost, or outcomes between Columbia nurse practitioners and physicians.

We established, and still run profitably 15 years later, the only independent nurse practitioner practice where commercial insurers (UnitedHealthcare, Aetna, and every other commercial insurers who accept Columbia physician billing) pay us the same rates as Columbia physicians (and in one instance that rate is higher than that of non-Columbia physicians). The practice, Columbia Advanced Practice Nurse Associates (CAPNA), is part of the Eastside Medical Practice for Columbia in midtown Manhattan at 60th Street and Madison Avenue. Several bold and brave chief executive officers (CEOs) of the major insurance companies were willing to profile our practices to their beneficiaries, even knowing the medical backlash they might incur.

This practice brought down the wrath of conservative medicine in New York State and in the nation. The American Medical Association (AMA) charged us with practicing medicine without a license; competing for commercial patients was the last straw for them, and we competed well. CBS, in a *60 Minutes* program narrated by Morley Safer, gave the public a stunningly positive view of CAPNA and depicted the AMA administrators who were so alarmed.

Building on this increasingly independent and publicly recognized model, we developed a degree program, which would incorporate the added skills and competencies nurses need to practice the full-scope, cross-site (office, hospital admitting and management, emergency room [ER] evaluations, on call) 24/7 responsibility. Existing nurse practitioner programs taught skills and competencies that were essentially limited to a single site (office or hospital-based practice). With the models we had developed, more knowledge was needed in the clinical realm, in informatics, and in how to run a business (which an independent practice most surely is).

This new Doctor of Nursing Practice (DNP) degree met with predictable skepticism in nursing, which recognized the enormity of what we were doing but did not have the same 10-year development of faculty with the required skills. Medical skepticism remained strong, but new degrees are the purview of a profession, not the public. We had our first graduates in 2005, and today, 8 years later, nearly every university-based nursing school in the country has, or is planning, a DNP program.

Knowing the new skills and knowledge needed to deliver this sophisticated care, we moved quickly to begin developing standards for the new degree. "Degree creep" is rampant in academics, and we worried that well-meaning but inadequately prepared schools could rename an MS degree as a DNP degree without their students achieving the same level of practice necessary for independent functioning in this new comprehensive care.

Again, as with the randomized controlled trial and with our commercial partners, we aimed for the highest standard we could achieve. In order to set a standard for the new DNP, we wanted one standard. We sought to do this by developing a certification program, whereby the successful test takers would have a national distinction showing insurers and patients that they had met the highest level of competence. We did this by partnering with the National Board of Medical Examiners (NBME), the premier testing organization in medicine. They agreed to develop a test for DNPs that would test the same competency as the final exam did for medical students to qualify for an MD degree. We were thrilled and knew the public would understand this certification. Obviously, the conservative medical profession once again roared and complained but, once again, we had a strong CEO (Don Melnick, MD, at the NBME) to back us up.

The next step was to have our new certification program approved by the national accrediting body, the Institute for Clinical Evaluation. This was accomplished as well, and so those who take the NBME exam for DNPs can use the certification to meet all nursing requirements for certification in advanced practice.

This story has significance far beyond nursing. It is a story of physician heroes at Columbia, the Columbia trustees, CEOs at Presbyterian Hospital, insurance companies, the NBME, the editor in chief of *JAMA*, and the 10 brave physicians from across the country who signed on the *JAMA* article after serving to help us conduct the trial.

This is also a story about how Columbia leaders (president, provost, legal affairs) from the central university responded to these innovations, how they handled our academic requests, and how they dealt with the media outpouring and the national campaign against nursing taking a higher role in American medicine.

The story has political significance, touching on universal access and other parts of the jeopardized health care plan under review. It is about how health policy is made and how innovations succeed if managed carefully.

Mary O'Neil Mundinger, DrPH, FAAN

• • • • •

Acknowledgment

• • • • •

VARTAN GREGORIAN

MANY WONDERFUL FRIENDS AND COLLEAGUES lifted me along the path of my 25 years as dean, but only one implored me to write about it. He said, "You must tell your story, because if you do not, someone else will, and you won't like it." So here is that story. My friend Vartan Gregorian is responsible for this book, because without his encouragement it would not have been written. For this and countless other times when he advised and gave me strength, I give him my thanks and my gratitude.

• • • • •

Tibetan Words and Symbols

• • • • •

As I wrote this tale of 25 years at the Columbia University School of Nursing, it seemed to be all action, conflict, and success. I was struck by how two-dimensional it appeared; but our experiences were far more than that. I wanted to convey the underlying perspectives and growing awareness of what we were achieving. I chose to use the Tibetan golden fish symbol, and the Tibetan alphabet to introduce the dedication and each subsequent section of this story. The Tibetan people provide a living example of the fortitude, perseverance, and courage it has taken to sustain their culture and community in Northern India and in the world. I hoped the third and lasting dimension of what we were attempting to accomplish, with unity and purpose, would be a reflection of how they, the Tibetan people, have so endured.

COVER—SUCCESS ལམ་ཆོང་།

This history of 25 years of challenge looks like an EKG tracing; radical and repeated upswings and downswings, with far more ups than downs. It is a story of success, won with great effort, joyous accomplishments, and the making of many lasting friendships.

DEDICATION—GOLDEN FISHES

The pair of golden fish is a sacred Buddhist icon. It is an auspicious sign, meaning life and happiness, fertility and abundance, conjugal fidelity, and unity. My husband Paul brought me all of these gifts, and most of all, love. He was my best friend.

A PATH TO EXCELLENCE—AWAKENING གྲུང་པོ་བཟོ་བྱེད། མིག་འབྱེད།

All the years of my career before my deanship at Columbia were filled with experiences, observations, mistakes, and the ever-present faith in me from my parents, my husband, and my colleagues. Only when I held a position where I had the authority to bring about great and good change could I understand how my "awakening" as a leader had been so carefully nurtured.

SECTION I—CRISIS དཀའ་རྙོག

The first 5 years of this quarter century of progress were filled with crises. Would the university close the school? Would the hospital take us over? Would the faculty have the courage and know-how to develop new academic and practice patterns? Could we turn around our financial deficits?

SECTION II— COURAGE སྙིང་སྟོབས།

In this 5-year time span—the early 1990s—we conducted the first randomized controlled trial (RCT) comparing nurse practioner (NP) practice with MD practice in primary care of Medicaid patients. Even more courageously, the NPs in the study learned and established new, more sophisticated skills caring for their patients across sites of care. This was necessary in order to match the authority of the MDs with whom they would be compared. Their MD colleagues stood by them, taught them, and helped them achieve these new levels of care—they too had courage: Red badges all around.

SECTION III—STRENGTH དཔུང་ཤུགས།

In the last half of the 1990s the depth of our new model was becoming apparent. We concluded the RCT with stunning results: there were no differences between NP and MD practice in cost, utilization, outcomes, or patient satisfaction. On the strength of these findings we opened a primary care practice for commercially insured patients: Columbia Advanced Practice Nurse Associates (CAPNA). Without the RCT results, and without our stalwart MD colleagues, our new practice could have faltered under the withering attack from organized medicine, which woke up to the competitive scope of practice we were introducing. Physicians had never opposed NPs caring for poor or underserved patients, but our bold mainstream endeavor hit at their finances in a new and potentially competitive way, which caused their rage and entitlement. The strength of our practice model— acknowledgment from payers who had too few primary care providers in their network—and the ever strong support of Columbia physicians made our new practice a success.

SECTION IV— CONFIDENCE ཡིད་ཆེས།

In the first 5 years of the new millennium we published the RCT results. We then began dual efforts to formalize the new learning and skills into a doctoral degree program in practice, and to convince our wary and conservative university that our idea would be adopted by other top-tier universities. Our president was so confident of our plan that he allowed us to develop a DNP curriculum and to enroll 17 of our faculty in the first program while the proposal to formally establish the new degree was wending itself through the university approval process. These two intermingled efforts took us 5 years.

SECTION V—HARMONY སྟུན་པོ། སྒྲ་མཐུནས་སྙིག་པོ།

The final 5 years of my leadership at Columbia were defined by a sense of harmony in what we had built together. We were "combining into a consistent whole" (*Webster's Third International Dictionary*) the practice phenomena, our pathbreaking health policy research program, and our innovative new degrees. We were, in a larger sense for our profession, "assuring the supremacy of the good" (*Webster's Third International Dictionary*), a rather imperious statement that nonetheless reflected our approach as we strove to build a fully autonomous and unique identity for nursing.

SECTION VI—EXCELLENCE ཕུལ་དུ་བྱུང་བ།

Excellence is defined as "the state of possessing good qualities in an eminent degree" (*Webster's Third International Dictionary*). Certainly this is a characteristic of leadership. Without such qualities in a leader, there is less to follow, or to emulate, or to improve. Progress always requires stepping on the shoulders of a predecessor; the stronger the shoulders, the higher and more certain the reach. We all owe each other that clear and stable base to move our followers ahead and past us. This, too, is excellence.

• • • • •

The Path to Excellence:
A Letter From the Author

• • • • •

ཀྱང་པོ་བརྗེ་བྱེད། མེག་འབྱེད།

REFLECTING ON MY LONG CAREER, it is clear that I always had an affinity for leadership. I'm sure it was in my nature, or in my DNA, but those nascent directives bloomed only when certain experiences were made available to me, and when certain individuals provided nurture and acknowledgment that I was on the right path. Leadership skills can be learned, but it requires certain personal characteristics to be successful. One has to have confidence and optimism and the ability to climb out of failures or mistakes without being too scared to dust oneself off and resume a hopeful path.

Because of the innovations and progress in nursing practice that were accomplished under my leadership at Columbia, many people view me as a visionary. A visionary—to me—has a far-off view of what should be and works tirelessly to achieve it. In that simple definition, I did have a vision: nursing in its most sophisticated presence, deserves recognition—and authority—as an independent profession. But I have lots of company from like-minded colleagues. Perhaps we are all visionaries within that broad definition, but the paths we have taken toward that goal are varied. I did not have a set of steps to be taken or a plan of sequential achievements. The randomized controlled trial (RCT) research comparing nurse practitioners (NPs) and medical doctors (MDs), the Columbia Advanced Practice

Nurse Associates (CAPNA) model, the clinical Doctor of Nursing Practice (DNP) degree, the American Board of Comprehensive Care (ABCC) certification, —all of these happened as a consequence of context. These successful steps each built on the preceding one—the RCT gave credibility to CAPNA, CAPNA became the DNP model, the ABCC exam gave nurses evidence of comparability to MD practice in comprehensive care—and all of this was fostered by the sustained deficit of primary care physicians, the context of our advancements in nursing. What we did was to act as courageous opportunists, not simply as visionaries. We were activists and not just dreamers.

And there was no grand plan. Each step in the progression of practice authority was taken for its own inherent value in advancing nursing, but I don't think any of us knew where it would ultimately go—and we still don't. Nursing's march toward recognition and value is still underway. But it took leadership and careful observation of the environment to make each step secure and meaningful.

In 1955, I was an 18-year-old college freshman, 380 miles from home, just weeks after the unexpected death of my beloved father from a heart attack. Cardiology was in its infancy then—reading EKGs was a new skill—but seeing the tracing of a damaged heart led only to bed rest and hope. No aspirin, no angioplasty, no grafts, no medicines. At 51, he had gone, and at 44, my bereft mother was alone with my 15-year-old brother. It was not an easy transition to college, and overnight I had lost my father and resources. I felt unanchored and poor, even though I was given financial aid, and I needed to find a part-time job to help fund my expenses. I began in the kitchen of my dorm, first as a prep dishwasher, separating the dirty dishes, glasses, and silverware into separate baskets and pushing them on the conveyor into the huge dishwasher. It wasn't heavy work, but it was steamy and tiring. I worked about 10 meals a week at first and, with the new minimum wage of 75 cents an hour, I made enough to meet my simple needs. By the end of the fall semester, I added more hours as I became comfortable with my academic schedule. Male students from other dorms were hired to wash the dishes, and carry the heavy trays of food to the serving area. By November, I had become smitten with one these coworkers, a tall, handsome, unpretentious senior, and although we hadn't even spoken, I made sure there were empty seats at the table I chose when all of us workers ate together before the doors opened for the students. When he finally asked me out, I of course said yes. But I already had a date for that night. I don't know why I didn't simply break the original date, but I didn't. The day arrived and I was filled with anxiety about how I was going to pull this off. At that time, there were no phones in the dorm rooms. There was a buzzer system; one buzz meant I had a visitor, and two buzzes meant my roommate had a visitor. When the buzzer went off—once—I went downstairs in trepidation that the wrong man had arrived, but as luck would be with me throughout my life, the person waiting for me was Paul. I don't know what happened when my originally scheduled date appeared. I was on a different path already.

As I began my sophomore year, I had a straight-A average and was loving my nursing courses. I was working about 20 hours a week on the food line and was thrilled that I could take my electives in the English department. As an undergraduate, Paul had taken an English course on Shakespeare, had found the professor incredibly good, and thought I should take the course. G.B. Harrison was the preeminent Shakespearean scholar then. Being an Englishman, he gave Shakespeare a voice that we will never forget. In a current blog remembering Harrison, one student from the 1960s wrote that "students were so in awe of him that none of us would talk to him."

That's not quite true. I couldn't wait to talk to him. I attended classes in my blue-and-white-striped nylon nursing uniform. Class was usually on a day in which I also had clinical hours at the hospital, and although I am sure there was time to change clothes, it never occurred to me that the English majors with whom I attended class might look down on me if I appeared as a nursing student. I took it for granted that nurses were smart people, and I was so secure in my career choice that it took me years to understand the conventional views of nurses as being merely doctors' helpers.

I took a second class from Professor Harrison in the spring, and part way through he asked me to meet with him. I showed up as usual in my nursing uniform not quite knowing what to expect. He told me I had an unusually good grasp of the material and wrote very well, and he asked if I would consider becoming an English major in the honors program. I was nonplussed and deeply touched. My father had loved his English courses at the University of Michigan in the late 1920s and was an inspired writer as well as successful businessman, and here I was following in his footsteps. I was eager to consider this opportunity, although it was an entirely new idea. Yes, I loved nursing, but here was a famous person telling me I might have the makings of a writer. Paul and I talked it over. The next year—my junior year—I would receive $100 a month from the university as a sign of my growing contribution to clinical care in the hospital. The first 2 years we students weren't worth much, but by our junior year we would be spending over 20 hours a week in lightly supervised bedside care. Paul and I were already thinking about getting married that summer, and $100 a month was a lot of money. Reluctantly I turned down Professor Harrison's offer. I never learned to be the writer I might have been, nor did I immerse myself in English literature scholarship, but I made the right choice, as my life with Paul and each decade in my life has proven. Harrison's comments, however, gave me great confidence in my writing and analytical skills. I would find that both could enhance my leadership style and what I could accomplish.

In the spring of my sophomore year I was 19 years old, and I was promoted in the dining hall to supervisor. I now had an office—a cubicle really, but private, with a desk. I was in charge of scheduling the student personnel and overseeing their work. I liked the administrative work and found I could work nearly 40 hours a week and still get 30 hours of clinical and class completed; in 1956, my pay nearly doubled to $1.42 an hour. We felt rich.

My junior year flew by. I was working in the kitchen or in the hospital nearly all the time. My supervisory job was increasingly fun for me, as I learned how the whole venture worked, including the adult, nonstudent, staff who became my friends, and colleagues, and learned how food was ordered and paid for. Paul and I became friends with the dishwasher who scrubbed the cooking pans and cleaned the stoves. He was an older man who loved literature, and we talked about Shakespeare. As my junior year ended, the dishwasher left, but not before he told us he was a writer and had been working as a dishwasher only to gather material for his next book, about the lowly workers in a big university. The book was called *Beetles in the Ivy*.

In August, during my 4-week vacation, Paul and I were married. Paul received his MS in that spring of 1958 and took a job with the Fish and Wildlife Service, while I completed my senior year. It was the beginning of over 50 years of his own field and lab research studying avian communications.

While Michigan nursing was extraordinarily ahead of its time in how nursing students were integrated into the university and given freedom with their personal lives, there were also many traditional accoutrements of our conservative profession. Caps differed widely, from those that looked like a cupcake wrapper to wide-winged contraptions that limited movement in and out of curtained bedsides. Michigan's cap was somewhere in between, a modest triangle. First-year students didn't merit any cap at all, but sophomores got a plain white one, juniors could add a thin black velvet stripe, and seniors—and graduates—a wide black velvet stripe. Black stripes on caps apparently signified a nurse's part in relieving suffering. Uniforms, too, were strictly designed to represent different years of education. This terribly structured and militaristic depiction of nursing was offensive to me. It placed nurses in a category of supervised workers. While proud of the addition of that first black stripe on my cap (I think we all like acknowledgment), I was uncomfortable with the whole system. It seemed to overly constrain nurses, as though they might exceed their authority without the visible signs of their limited professional status. It simply galled me.

In 1959, I graduated, and Paul had been accepted for PhD study at Cornell. We left for Ithaca, with me 7 months pregnant. I took a position at Tompkins County Hospital and was assigned to the obstetrics department. My best friend from age 9, Pat Black, had also gone to Michigan with me, was married to a Cornell Vetenary School student, and was hired in the same obstetrics department. We were also both terrified. Our Michigan experience had been extensive in obstetrics, overseen by Hazel Avery (Miss Ovary is what we called her, of course), but we hadn't ever been in charge of a labor and delivery suite, nor had we had experienced determining the stage of labor of a patient. In a medical center, that was done by medical residents; in Ithaca, though, this was our responsibility. We were totally unprepared for this role. I can still remember the overwhelming anxiety I felt on the days I was assigned to the labor and delivery unit; the postpartum and newborn nursery assignments were fun and easy, but labor and delivery was another story. There were three delivery rooms and five labor rooms, plus the hallway in between, which we often needed for laboring patients, with one nurse and one aide. A lot was expected of us as University of Michigan graduates; there were very few nurses with bachelor's degrees at the hospital, but the other nurses let us know how inadequate we were. I don't think we let on how uneasy we were in the labor suite, but there was no hiding the fact that we didn't know how to put together an instrument tray or work the autoclave.

Not only was the hospital not staffed by residents, but the attending physicians weren't around all the time either. During the day, they had full-time office hours, some in solo practices, and they all wanted to be home, sleeping, at night. We nurses were in charge. One physician piloted his own glider on weekends. There were no cell phones then, so if the physician had a patient in labor, and if in my heightened intuitive fright I decided that his patient was close to delivery, I would call his wife, and she would move their car out of the garage into the driveway as a signal to her husband, gliding by, to land and go to the hospital. I was always mindful that it would not go over well if I interrupted his weekend respite with a false alarm. But I didn't want to deliver a baby either. I was haunted by the possibility of a breech or shouldering the delivery on my own. The majority of our patients were Cornell students having their first babies, which only worsened my concerns over my competence. And I was doing all of this in the last 8 weeks of my own first pregnancy; I knew full well that I could end up in the hands of a wide-eyed nurse like me who didn't know what was going on. Pat and I learned quickly; we often had more than six births a day, and she was with me as my nurse when I had my baby.

Fathers then were not allowed in the labor suite, nor were they allowed to embrace or even touch their baby. But all of a sudden we were three. And the difference was profound.

I returned to work full time in 6 weeks, working the evening shift, and Paul scheduled all of his classes and lab work to allow him to be with our son while I was at work. He would read and rock the baby carriage with his foot, keeping our son quiet and sleeping while he studied. When I got home, he would go off to bed, little Paul would wake up, and it would be 1 or 2 a.m. before I went to bed. This schedule, however, was not as tandem as it appeared. By January, I was pregnant with our second child.

During those months I became confident of my role in the labor suite. I got better at determining when labor was coming to the point of delivery, but I never was given the opportunity to learn to do clinical examinations that gave me measurable approximations of a woman's progress. I simply learned to assess by her reactions to what was going on inside her, and that exquisite ability to see nuanced responses was instrumental in my growing ability to read her thinking and attitudes and proclivities. It was an invaluable training in observation that informed my administrative responsibilities and political acumen 25 years later, when I was given the dean position. It was also an unparalleled opportunity to bring policy to bear on the very issues that would advance nursing.

In these early years of my career, I was practicing in an environment without an academic presence, where research and medical and nursing training was absent. It was all about clinical care. In the labor suite we were a small group of professionals working closely together. I learned to give anesthesia, how to resuscitate a newborn and how to—eventually on New Year's Eve—deliver babies—even a breech on my own. When we were busy, there were more physicians than nurses. We were all on a first-name basis, which I accepted as a natural and good thing. When I later stumbled on the conventionality of more conservative environments, I saw no need to accept that view; I had successfully experienced another way of interacting. Once I became confident of my abilities in the labor suite it was where I preferred to be. I liked the pace, the decisions I could make, and the drama. I liked running things, just as I had at Michigan—only now I was in the hospital, not the dining room. I was on my way.

I have always held nursing practice in great esteem; I see it as the core of our profession. It informs our research and our teaching, even when not directly linked. For example, in teaching health policy, it is imperative that public policy makers fully understand the value of nursing's unique contributions (as well as its helper role) without which the "team" would be lacking a critical component. In researching health care informatics, as another example, it is crucial that the language and observations specific to nursing be incorporated in the coding and analysis. Nursing practice is the often invisible—or discounted—element of advancing the health of individuals, and we need our own best practitioners to tell their stories. This is what was driving me in 1998 when we developed centers that would give equal access to clinicians and researchers to participate, and when I made sure that we established endowed chairs for clinicians as well as researchers. During the 1995–2000 years, three of the four endowed chairs, Gill, Pettit, and Irving, were established for clinical professors. It is rare indeed—and perhaps nowhere at all—that a nontenured faculty member could be appointed to an endowed chair in a major university. We wanted to change that and give equal recognition to our bright and system-changing clinical faculty. In the next 5 years, we would take this plan one important step further, in developing the first doctoral degree in the world for advanced and sophisticated nurse clinicians, and in endowing two more chairs for clinical scholars.

All four of our children were born in Ithaca, and when Paul finished his doctorate, we moved to Miami University in Oxford, Ohio. I worked evenings at the local hospital, where nurses were in short supply. I was in charge of labor and delivery, the pharmacy, and the emergency room (ER). One night when I was caring for a woman in labor, a horrendous car accident occurred, and four teenagers arrived in the ER. One died. The other three needed urgent care. It was a terrible situation, and I was filled with fear that I might not be able to provide what they—and my labor patient—needed before physician help arrived. Afterward I resigned my nursing position because I couldn't accept the deep lack of nursing staff. I knew I had to find a place in nursing where I had the authority to make things happen in a high-quality way.

I turned my attention to raising money for an outdoor skating rink. We had loved watching Cornell hockey in Ithaca (Paul had been the team's academic advisor) and I thought it would be wonderful to start a junior hockey program in Oxford. I raised the money—$5,000—which may not seem noteworthy except it rarely ever got below freezing in Oxford. This was my first fundraising effort, and I liked doing it.

We left Miami after a year when Paul was awarded a postdoctoral fellowship at the Rockefeller University in New York City. We moved to Rye and I found myself once again working at the local hospital, but this time on a day shift, since our children were now all in school. I gave a few presentations to the nursing staff on the emerging area of nursing diagnosis. This idea piqued my interest because I saw it as a tool of distinguishing, and advancing, nursing practice. I became a zealot on the idea, and the nursing director appointed me head of the inservice education department, in charge of recruitment and training. The first thing I did was to design and give a course to the nurse aides so that they could do more for patients, including taking vital signs and monitoring the pace of IV infusions, for example. We offered them a certificate as an advanced nurse aide. They were so proud, and the nurses were grateful. We made a big deal about the skills and standards the certifications represented.

Meanwhile I began contributing to a national group of nurses who were further refining nursing diagnosis, and I published my first paper in one of nursing's leading journals. Having been sold on the idea that nurses could, within their domain, make diagnoses about health problems that nurses could treat, I was struck by the fact that there was no system in place that would ensure that the nurse's diagnosis and plan of care would be carried out. We needed a new system whereby a nurse who was trained to make nursing diagnoses would have the authority to make sure the plan of care and evaluations would be followed on every shift and that the authorized nurse would have continuity with the patients receiving this care. Until then, nurses were randomly assigned on each shift; one might or might not care for the same patients on successive days, and every nurse could daily decide what nursing care to give, in addition to the care designed and ordered by a physician.

Giving nursing diagnosis a chance to succeed meant changing the system of delivering nursing care. We did that at this little hospital and called it Primary Nursing. As we built the standards for who could be a primary nurse, in charge of a continuing group of patients and responsible for designing and directing nursing care based on nursing diagnoses, the role took on great luster. We believed a nurse with the new authority should be a full-time employee. In short order, the department was overwhelmed with requests from nurses to obtain full-time instead of part-time status. We held courses and developed a curriculum and competencies for a primary nurse. We awarded certificates to those who met the new standards.

This evolution had two interesting outcomes. One, full-time employees got benefits and they got higher salaries, making this new program a costly one for the hospital. Part-time nurses rarely made as much per day as a full-time nurse, and they received no benefits. The other outcome was more profound. Primary nurses took their responsibilities seriously, and developed great pride and assertiveness regarding their practice. They demanded more staff when it was needed, and they expected physicians to treat them differently, since they now shared responsibilities for the same given patients, over time. The physicians had not been paying attention to our advancements and were annoyed by the newly empowered nurses. I vividly remember trying to convince a surgeon that a nursing diagnosis related to a patient's anxiety was worth addressing with a plan of education and support for the patient and his family. He simply saw no reason for these time-consuming nursing endeavors and said to me in deep frustration, "Damn it, the anxiety will go away when he goes home. Just do what I want done." But the momentum in nursing—at our hospital and nationally—was moving to develop primary nursing as a quality initiative in many hospitals.

Within the next year, the hospital employed the Ernst and Ernst firm to study its efficiency. With the hospital's finances in trouble, the new president thought inefficiencies needed to be addressed. The outcome of that study caused a huge conflagration at the hospital. The chief of surgery, chief of staff, and chief of medicine were fired from their administrative positions in response to their written demands regarding patient safety issues. Primary nursing was deemed too expensive: one article in the local paper reported that the study had described many nursing activities as "niceties, such as teaching a newly discovered diabetic how to administer his or her medication after leaving the hospital." The director of nursing and the three assistant directors (including me) were fired. Public uproar ultimately caused the board to fire the president of the hospital, whose idea it had been to conduct the efficiency study. The hospital dismantled the primary nursing system, and new leaders were recruited. Several years later, the hospital closed its doors for good, as the financial deficits were never resolved.

In my journal in 1977, when I was fired, I described the uncertainty of what I should do next. I wanted to reinvent primary nursing somewhere else, but I wrote, "I know that the future for professional nursing isn't in the inpatient setting. I want to be in ambulatory care—I don't just want to be in it, I want to direct it. The nurses must be full practitioners, with all the physical data–gathering skills. I'll need them too if I'm to be a believable director." I took a position as an assistant professor at Pace University so that I could be in the first cohort to train faculty nurse practitioners, a certificate program for Pace faculty.

During this time I wrote my first book, *Autonomy in Nursing*. It was a series of case studies on sites of care where nurses practice and on the systems they used in those settings to implement their growing independent authority. Primary nursing was front and center for inpatient nursing, and nurse practitioner was the ambulatory model. I wrote that skills and knowledge, not site of care, determined autonomy.

After completing my nurse practitioner training, I was accepted in the health policy department as a doctoral student at Columbia's School of Public Health. I raced through the program in 2 years because I saw how instrumental such a degree would be in my crusade to develop independent practice policies for nursing. My dissertation explored how public health nurses implemented Medicare's home health policies. It was the basis for my second book, *Home Care Controversy: Too Little, Too Late, Too Costly*. Much of my analysis included the flaws in the Medicare law and described nurses' attempts to give care that was needed, even when not allowed under the statute. My observations were that nursing direction of home care (without the more focused medically oriented requirements) would have resulted in better health and lower costs. Although policy oriented, rather than being descriptions of practice, the two books had a similar tone and approach: there is a fundamental gap in the health care system that can be filled by recognizing nurses' authority to direct and deliver the care they are competent to provide. In many ways, this present book is a continuation of the same thinking and beliefs. In each stage of development—identifying the health problems nurses independently resolve (nursing diagnoses), specifying the inpatient system needed to operationalize that authority (primary nursing), observing how nurses in a variety of roles and settings can independently assess and give care and now awarding the clinical doctorate and competency certification to assure the public that these nurses deserve independent authority in health care—the same overriding value shines through: Nurses are autonomous, valuable, and distinctive resources in health care. Nurses stand alone in their elegant, unique, and fundamental contributions to the health and well-being of their patients.

Although this year-by-year picture of my professional accomplishments may appear to have been center stage in my life, it was not. I enjoyed the rare and precious support of my husband as my professional responsibilities grew, and I found great joy in his equally vibrant and consuming interests, and in our strong, close family. Because so much of what I attempted and engaged in was radical and outside the norm, I would have been viewed as either a mere dilettante or a zealot if I wasn't most importantly and most fundamentally a conventional wife and mother. My husband anchored my path-breaking ideas through his grounded intellect, calm wisdom, sure love and support, and his pride in what I was doing. Without him and his belief in me, I would not have had the courage or the power to do what I did.

It's easy to think I was a clear-minded standard-bearer, with a vision of where I was headed in my career, but that was not the case. I had a broad vision, not a detailed one, and I was an opportunist, seeing where we might go as time and events gave us openings and leverage. My freedom to devote myself to these possibilities came from Paul. While he was developing his own productive and imaginative research, he always had time to be with me, and through his presence and personal credibility, he enhanced mine. The achievements described in this book are dedicated to him.

Section I

• • • • •

Survival—The Ultimate Challenge: 1985–1990

• • • • •

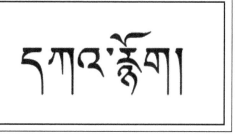

1
•••••

Avoiding Failure

•••••

ARRIVING AT COLUMBIA AS AN assistant professor in 1983, the year before I left for my Robert Wood Johnson Foundation health policy fellowship in Washington, DC, I learned for the first time the history of the school's nursing program. Joann Jamann, appointed the first school leader as a full academic dean in 1981, was also the first doctorally prepared head of the school and the first nonalumna in that position. Unfortunately, however, she failed to fully engage the faculty or the alumni and got caught up in the national nursing educational downturn and financial meltdown of the school, and so she resigned in 1985. I was the second nonalumna leader, and the first dean married with children. Although my career mirrors that of many of my dean colleagues elsewhere—married with children, career positions in many institutions (rarely were any of us appointed to positions in our alma mater)—I was nonetheless an oddity at Columbia Nursing where all but my immediate predecessor and Mary Crawford, who had a short dual role as director of hospital nursing and the school, were alumni who were hospital nurses and school administrators at the medical center for their entire careers. This pattern had held for nearly 100 years. I don't believe any other current university school had such a narrow and parochial history of its leaders. This does not negate the brilliance and devotion of many of these women, but clearly they had no other context for leadership than what they had experienced as nurses and faculty at Presbyterian Medical Center. This may be part of the reason for the delayed independence of the nursing school and the lack of foresight in the 1970s when the school could have forestalled the academic and financial problems of the early 1980s. Indeed, when Columbia's main campus was in wild disarray with the 1968 student riots, the nursing students uptown were still peacefully marking their transition into their second year of study by hanging black stockings out their dorm windows as a statement that, as upper-class students, they had earned the right to wear white stockings. It was indeed a time warp.

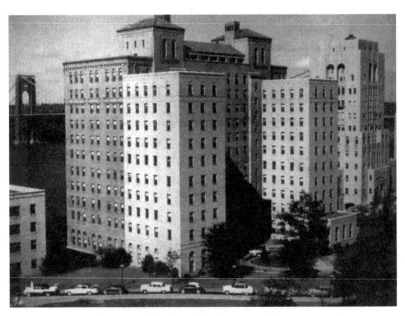

Maxwell Hall as it looked in 1950.

● ● ● ● ●

The nursing school was immune to the world changing around it during these immutable years. The nurses dutifully wore the right uniform (and stockings), stood when a physician arrived in the hospital ward, and followed the time-honored rules that were fast disappearing in other university schools of nursing. Columbia's nursing students were then—as they are now—among the best-educated clinicians in the world. They accomplished these goals early on in an atmosphere that was decades out of date. Without experience in other university settings, it is not surprising that Columbia nursing leaders kept doing what the person before them had done, and the school fell gravely out of step with how modern schools nursing function. But for all those years they had occupied the premier building of the medical center, and now it was gone. Learning the history of the school during those long years helped me understand how the school had arrived at its perilous position and also understand the deep legacy attached to Maxwell Hall.

This historic first building of the medical center, housing 19 stories of offices, classrooms, and dormitory for the School of Nursing since 1927, had a magnificent lobby with a grand piano, a rooftop with a stunning view of the Hudson River, and a large indoor swimming pool was gone. This had replaced Florence Nightingale Hall in midtown where the nursing school was established and where the medical school had been located

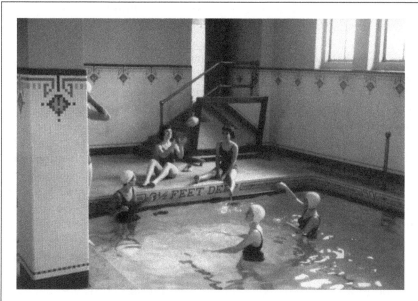

Maxwell Hall pool in 1965.

● ● ● ● ●

when a constellation of hospitals—Babies, Neurological Institute, and Presbyterian—moved to Washington Heights, the nursing school was the first to claim a spot and build a building in the newly established medical center. It cost $1 million and the alumni paid for it. No credit was given to the school when the building came down because the alumni donors had graduated from Presbyterian Hospital School of Nursing and the hospital claimed the building as theirs in 1982 when it was demolished. They built a physicians' office building on the site. The school was relocated to two floors in the Georgian Building, which had been built in the 1920s as a dorm for medical residents.

I returned from Washington in the fall of 1985 to a new position in the Office of Vice President for Health Sciences, headed by Dr. Henrik Bendixen. The enrollment in the School of Nursing had dropped 50% in the previous 3 years, from 346 to 178. The school was in arrears to the university for almost $1 million ($914,000), which it would have to pay back from its small endowment of $2 million. The majority of administrative positions were vacant; communications with prospective students and governmental, financial, and organizations were late, absent entirely, or inaccurate. The school had 35 full-time faculty, two of whom were involved in (unfunded) research, and none were engaged in practice. I refused to return to this sinking ship and therefore was offered the position in Bendixen's office.

In response to the school's budget proposal submitted in 1985, Provost Robert Goldberger wrote Dean Jamann:

Your budget submission outlines a plan of action during which we all agree will be several difficult years for the School of Nursing. Given the many financial pressures the school is facing, the poor prospects for federal support of nursing research, the number of doctoral programs already competing for those funds. . . .

In that same summer of 1985, the new president of Presbyterian Hospital, Dr. Thomas Morris, in a meeting with university administration, outlined his thoughts on medical center nursing: "unifying hospital and university nursing in one person assures the best use of joint resources." He suggested using the hospital-based associate degree program (The Clark School) as the first 2 years toward earning BS and MS degrees at Columbia. He believed this would allow "normal turf concerns to disappear and new ideas to be tried." He was essentially suggesting that Columbia students begin their education in a hospital-based associate degree program where they could first become registered nurses (RNs) before pursing higher degrees. Morris, a distinguished internist, had spent his entire career at Columbia often "acting" in various administrative positions and possessing great gravitas in the medical community. As hospital president, he exerted his beliefs strongly for the first time—conventionally rooted in his long-held respect for the hospital. Having weathered the wrenching transition from hospital to university in 1937, the nursing school was still considered a subset of the medical school in 1986, nearly 50 years later. Morris's rescue proposal in the summer 1985 would place the school once again within the hospital structure. In the 1986 competitive climate for nursing students, this old and outdated theme spelled professional and financial ruin for our fine school.

Two years earlier, in a December 23, 1983, letter from Bob Levy, then vice president for Health Sciences, to Edward Norian, executive vice president of the Presbyterian Hospital, plans for full occupancy of the Georgian Building by the School of Nursing were laid out in a legal memo of understanding. Nearly 30 years later the school was still only a partial occupant of the Georgian Building and without its own home. The school was not a priorty in the medical center or at the university.

When I returned to Columbia in the fall of 1985, one of my projects in Bendixen's office was to analyze the status of the School of Nursing, particularly its financial and academic resources. In December, as the school continued its disastrous unraveling, Bendixen relieved the current dean from her position. He determined that the school would close unless I agreed to take a limited 2-year deanship in a concentrated effort and ambitious plan to plant the seeds for renewal. Bendixen and Dr. William Hubbard, then chairman of the University Trustee Committee on the Health and Sciences, pledged their support for what would be a major challenge not only to turn the school around, but to convince the provost and the university that the school should be allowed to succeed.

I led the school for more than 20% of its long 118-year history, and more than half of all alumni graduated during this period. The major challenges I faced were the same as those of my predecessors, and perhaps were similar to those who follow me. First is its standing as an academic presence in the university, second is the tortured relationship between hospital and university nursing, and third is how professional nursing can distinguish itself in the eyes of the public when the vast majority of its members do not even hold a baccalaureate degree. Interestingly and provocatively, while the hospital leadership could never give up trying to capture the school within its own limited domain, Columbia physicians have never been a barrier in these areas, although medicine conventionally and nationally has posed challenges to the rise of professional nursing. In part, I believe this is because Columbia School of Nursing has always focused on its clinical excellence, which resonates with physicians, and in part because Columbia physicians are among the most elite in their profession and have little need for hierarchical distinctions.

FIRST CHALLENGE

As I began my 2-year deanship on December 20, 1985, the university's overwhelming expectation was that the school must partner with Presbyterian Hospital Nursing and return to its hospital roots to survive. Three days later, in a letter dated December 23, 1985, Presbyterian Hospital president Thomas Morris wrote to his nursing and medical vice presidents about the future of the Columbia School of Nursing. He began: "During the last few weeks Dr. Bendixen has informed me that unless the Presbyterian Hospital and Columbia University can develop a mutually supportive program for education of nursing students under the BS degree program, Columbia will be obliged to close the school." Surprisingly, this was not the picture Bendixen had painted for me. He believed in nursing but had no firm vision of what it could be in a university. Dr. Bendixen expected me to develop that vision: This was my first challenge. Morris, who had spent his entire career at the medical center, was not sanguine that a partnership would work. "After reviewing the past 50 years of relationship and agreements regarding nursing education (at the medical center), I am rather dismayed." He went on to list 15 steps the hospital would require in order to partner with the school, including consideration of changing the name of the school to Columbia Presbyterian School of Nursing, continuing the hospital's associate degree program, taking students from other nursing schools for clinical experience at Presbyterian (although all Columbia students would be required to study only at Presbyterian) and developing a new, heavily hospital-oriented clinical education that would "necessitate a lengthening of the usual program," essentially staffing the hospital 30 hours a week, so that students would have to fit into a "staggering" of classes in order to staff the hospital, and paying Presbyterian nurses to be clinical educators. This was an alarming prospect.

The school began as a Presbyterian Hospital school in 1892. The relationship of the school and hospital had begun to fray significantly in 1937 when the university incorporated the Division of Nursing into the Medical School and offered a BS degree. The 45-year-old school was one of the last in the nation to move into a university and offer an academic degree. This move, and the rancor of the hospital, did not cease in 1937. This painful breach had not healed by 1986–1989 when the school's desperate finances offered the hospital an opportunity to reclaim the school's reliance and "training." Tom Morris, in 1987, even after our clear renewal had begun, wrote a letter to Bendixen describing his deep concern about the 50-year history—from 1936 to 1986—of "bad blood" between the hospital and the school of nursing.

Academic and hospital nursing disconnects were not the only ones in the long and often inflamed relationship between the hospital and the university; the hospital and medical school also have a long history of failed "partnerships." In an agreement dated September 29, 1922, the combination of the historic College of Physicians and Surgeons joined the collective of Presbyterian Hospital, Babies Hospital, and the Neurological Institute, with the financial beneficence of Edward S. Harkness, and the medical center took shape. These agreements between the hospital and medical school were amended at least seven times in the 48 years between 1922 and 1970. Still attempting to sustain both independence and partnership between the university and hospital, the 1970 agreement sets up a governing board for the medical center, with the president and six members from each organization, which would cogovern and jointly select a director of the medical center. That model, as did previous ones, did not survive, and today the hospital and university leadership remain separate. This dance of independent partnership has led to increasing distinctions as National Institutes of Health (NIH) grants and office-based practice revenues funded the academic endeavor. Nursing was simply a subset of this dissonance.

SECOND CHALLENGE

Another important challenge was hidden in Article 4 of the 1970 agreement between Columbia's medical school and Presbyterian Hospital. Amazingly, 23 years before becoming a reality, the 1970 document gave credibility to the 1993 granting of admitting privileges to nurse faculty members. Article 4, regarding admitting privileges, states, in its entirety, "the professional staffs of the Hospital are to be appointed by the Hospital on the nomination of the University and are to consist of professors and other members of the University Medical School *and of persons of comparable professional standing*" (italics added).

We met this challenge through our single achievement in 1993: demonstrating that our clinical faculty had "comparable professional standing." This was and remains one of the most important accomplishments of my tenure as dean. It took many layers of achievement and recognition to build this recognition, and Columbia nurse researchers and clinicians were the brave, bold, and brilliant instruments of this extraordinary step forward for the profession. The opening for clinical advancement had been incorporated in a document 23 years earlier, at a time when no one in the medical center could have foreseen what this advancement might mean for nursing.

Hospital nursing had another arm to its presence in the nursing school: the Alumni Association. Although traditional alumni associations foster support for their school, the original Alumni Association for Columbia Nursing was entirely different. This Alumni Association was established not to support the school or its students, but rather to foster the welfare of its alumni. The association was further alienated from the school by being incorporated outside the university as a separate 501(c)3 and raising money in competition with the school. This strange entity was in part due to the times in which it was founded. In the late 1800s, nurses were primarily unmarried women bound to their profession, not unlike nuns in a religious order. Few nurses practiced after marriage. Fewer still had any pension or retirement benefits, even though they had practiced for decades after graduation. The Presbyterian Hospital Nursing School Alumni Association had a unique and noble mission: to care for its own. This, however, created a deep and artificially divisive fissure between the school and its future alumni. Even with its sole focus on alumni, the association has done very little on their behalf. With an endowment of $4 million in the 1980s, it donated only a few thousand dollars a year to alumni. In the perilous years of 1982–1986, when it looked like the school might fail, the Alumni Association was silent. I was not aware of the organization's existence until some months into my new role. Although Alumni Association benefits were small and rare (one needy alumnus was receiving checks of $13 per month), an annual meeting of alumni was their major activity. Dues of $25 a year allowed hundreds to easily join, and with few beneficiaries, their coffers grew so that their endowment in 1985 was more than double that of the school. In the painful next few years, a wary rapprochement was negotiated for the 1992 centennial, with the Alumni Association providing partial funding of two endowed chairs, and then a falling apart as Alumni Association leadership—those still in place from the 1950s—could not permanently breach the gap in mission.

THIRD CHALLENGE

Our third challenge, to provide the public with a clear and distinctive recognition of nursing at its most professional level, would be more easily met than the first two. This is where we would begin; the hospital and alumni challenges would have to wait—or be part of our devoted efforts to expand the reach of our profession. Underlying these challenges was the overwhelming need to develop financial stability for the school; our debts were greater than our income, and all of the potential sources of revenue were deeply eroded. In a survey I conducted shortly after taking the deanship, full-time faculty reported spending 2 ½ days a week on school responsibilities; clearly, productivity was an issue. Half of our tiny endowment was committed to paying our past debt, enrollments were dropping precipitously, the most promising faculty were leaving for stronger positions elsewhere, and the university and hospital viewed us as having only one alternative: becoming a clinical resource for the hospital. If we could find other sources of financial support to sustain and grow our independence, we could do so much more.

2
•••••

Faculty Practice: The Essential Cornerstone of Our Future
•••••

IT IS RARE INDEED, FOR students to have a nurse faculty member who is engaged in clinical care with authority at the highest level of their training. This is a major deficit for nursing students and for nursing schools. Students—even novices—very quickly intuit which faculty members know what they are teaching, and nursing faculty clinical experience is often decades old. Even for a diligent faculty member keeping up with clinical advancements, there is no substitute for having a faculty member fresh from his or her own clinical practice, arriving in the classroom to tell students what must be learned. The robust and sophisticated clinical teaching that arises from current experience is invaluable. In 1986 we believed this difference would enrich our student recruitment efforts.

But there were other reasons in addition to state of the art teaching that we wanted to address. Perhaps most immediate was the opportunity to unburden the school of excess faculty (too little productivity, too few students). If faculty would spend part of their work in salaried practice—say 50% of their time—then the school salary for that person would decrease by 50%. In this manner, we could drastically reduce the otherwise unnecessary terminations of surplus faculty. Such a model raised all kinds of questions. Could our faculty practice? Were they too far removed—in years and training—from engaging in a high-level practice? Although few of our faculty then had doctorates, all had master's degrees, but many of those degrees were in teaching or administration, not advanced practice. Those who were nurse practitioners, or midwives or clinical nurse specialists at least had a potential level of practice that would enrich our own advanced practice degree programs. But what about the others? Was there an appropriate clinical practice at a level that matched a BS educational level? What would a BS-prepared faculty "practice" if his or her master's degree was in education? While this disparity would be highly unusual in a university nurse faculty today, it was a challenge in 1986.

STRUCTURING THE FACULTY PRACTICE MODEL

In addition to finding the right site for practice that would fit the faculty member's expertise, we faced a major challenge in determining how to structure the financial aspects of the plan. First, we did not want to develop a model where a faculty member had two part-time jobs. We wanted faculty members to have one position, one set of benefits, and an aggregate salary that was at least equal to what their academic salary would otherwise be; this would preclude a practice that paid less than the faculty salary. If a faculty member made $40,000 at Columbia, but the practice available to him or her carried a full-time salary of $30,000, then someone practicing 50% of the time would only make a total of $35,000, which was unacceptable.

We also did not want a model whereby a faculty member might take on a small practice responsibility "moonlighting" for a salary that would supplement their full-time faculty salary; and we didn't want a model whereby faculty might "donate" a few hours a week to a clinical faculty. We wanted a fully accountable and integrated practice that carried academic weight and responsibilities, and an aggregate salary of the same or more than the faculty salary alone would yield.

In 1986, faculty salaries were somewhat higher than practice salaries (except perhaps in nurse anesthesia). As a result, we had to negotiate better salaries for faculty in the practice sites than others might earn in the same site for the same practice.

Another disparity was benefits. University benefits were better than nearly all the practice site benefits for employees. We developed our algorithm to make sure that each practice faculty had full university benefits, which became part of salary negotiations. We structured this new model to make it attractive to the faculty member. It worked, but it was messy and complicated and at the beginning it was confusing for everyone. Here is how we went through the process.

The new faculty practice group began meeting early in 1986, as did the other committees (low enrollment majors, precepting, research development). The committee was formed to develop a plan; they were charged with developing a definition of faculty practice, an analysis to learn about (or develop) several models, goals and objectives of the chosen plan, strategies for implementation, anticipated problems, and recommendations.

By the end of February, they had a model and had developed a time line and a list of pros and cons. Sarah Cook, who led this committee, showed the direct and collaborative leadership she would provide to the school for the next 25 years; she listened to all the concerns and then resolved as many as she could, always keeping the focus on developing a model that would benefit both faculty and the school and that would be marketable to practice sites. She came to be known as a wizard—a very popular one—by the faculty, who revered and trusted and loved her.

DEVELOPING THE FINANCIAL MODEL FOR FACULTY PRACTICE

The model they chose was to make practice a percentage of a full-time appointment (not additive), with full salary being the combination of school and practice salaries. Faculty appointment would remain full time in the school.

First, each clinical faculty member was evaluated in terms of how much of his or her time was required for faculty responsibilities. This might be 3 days a week. This left 2 days a week (40% of their time and salary) for practice. We were working on the assumption that a full-time faculty member was expected to be engaged 5 days a week. Once we knew what percentage of time was available for practice, faculty members had the responsibility to seek a clinical site where they wanted to practice. Our school developed a template for a faculty practice contract so that a faculty member could understand and agree to the financial, professional, and time commitments. We initially segregated faculty expenses between salary and fringe benefits, and we expected the clinical site to pay both to the school on behalf of the practitioner. For example, the university paid 30% of a faculty salary into the university's fringe benefit pool, which then paid for all of the benefits due to each faculty member (health insurance, contributions to their retirement account, subsidized parking, etc.). Therefore, the "cost" of each faculty member was salary plus 30% or more toward benefits. In order to ensure that a faculty member in practice would sustain full university benefits, we asked the potential practice site to prorate both costs in reimbursing the school. The school then took those dollars, placed the salary amount into the faculty member's paycheck, and the additional 30% into the fringe benefit pool, just as we did for every full-time faculty member. For instance, if a faculty salary was $40,000, it would actually cost the school $52,000, including the cost of benefits. If that faculty member was going to be half time in practice, we needed $26,000 from the site.

PROVIDING THE RATIONALE FOR CLINICAL SITES TO HIRE COLUMBIA FACULTY PRACTITIONERS

It came as a no surprise that clinical sites balked at this dual price tag. First of all, they could hire a part-time nurse for a lot less and had no responsibility for benefits. And with a part-time employee, there were no costs for benefits. Why on earth would they pay such a premium for a faculty practitioner? And why pay for benefits?

We learned to respond to these concerns in many ways, but fundamentally, we used the nursing shortage as our trump card. First, clinical sites could not attract and hire nurses with the caliber of our faculty for their clinical positions, especially not as part-time clinicians. With our faculty, they had a premier clinician who would bring with him or her a cadre of aspiring young nurses (students) who could be mentored by the faculty member while practicing. Those students, upon graduation, might be new recruits for the clinical site. If a site were to contract for two 50% faculty (a full-time equivalent), the site would have two experts for the price of one (albeit part time each) and money saved from their own benefit costs could be used to help pay university benefits for the two. This was a very confusing argument (though true), but we finally changed our contracts to require an aggregate dollar amount; internally at the school we separated out money for salary from money for benefits. The benefit cost was embedded in the one cost, and this one cost—though higher than the market price—was accepted. The school still split it up after receipt, with 30% going into the fringe benefit pool, but we no longer had two costs to support.

As the early Columbia providers began the process, the clinical sites were very pleased with the quality of their practice and the opportunity to recruit their students. Moreover, with time the differentiated cost of having a faculty practitioner became irrelevant. The major factor in this financial acceptance was the quality of the faculty in the clinical positions. The other mitigating factor was the presence of practitioners from the university's medical school in most of these clinical sites. It was generally acknowledged that university faculty in practice were elite and qualified, and brought extra value. We used the medical practice model, incorporating students, research colleagues, and state-of-the-art clinical practice. In many important ways, nursing practice came of age through faculty practice.

CREATIVELY NAVIGATING THE FACULTY PRACTICE MODEL

Although the financial model for faculty practice now sounds clear and precise, it was full of holes in the beginning. Payments to the school for faculty practice were often late or incorrect. Some sites persisted in sending checks directly to the practitioner, fracturing the "full-time" composite we had crafted. At times, the practice salary was not sufficient to cover the faculty salary, and the school tried to make accommodations that borrowed from school funds to pay a practice salary. Sometimes, too, a faculty member didn't fulfill all the required days of practice and the site dunned the school (appropriately). We learned how to divide sick days and vacation days prorata between the school and practice site; if the school's benefits were richer (more vacation days, for example), we had to account for that in the pro-rata division of benefits. It was a very complex process, and we were learning day by day how to titrate the dollars.

In addition to these issues we had to face a disparity between university and clinical site time frames. Faculty have significant time away from their formal responsibilities—Christmas break is weeks long, no one works on a holiday, the summer break may be 3 months or 1 month, depending on whether a faculty member taught in the summer session. This was not the case in a clinical site. Outpatient sites were more similar in terms of holidays and weekends, but hospital-based sites, even for advanced practice nurses, had a 24/7 rhythm of expectations. Faculty practitioners were quick to make these accommodations and even add to their salaries: if they had no summer academic responsibilities, they might increase their practice time (and income) at the very time those sites needed vacation replacement clinician care. More difficult were faculty who treasured their summers of free time, but now had a practice responsibility that was based on a 12-month commitment.

Nurses are very resourceful, and our faculty was no different. They began careful negotiations of their time commitments—full time instead of 50% for 6 weeks and then 6 weeks free of responsibilities, or they "banked" extra days by practicing more days during university holidays so that their summers were free. Once the financial model and days of practice per year were contracted, there was enough flexibility to develop satisfying practices.

In a May 1986 letter to faculty, I noted that every faculty member would have a partially subsidized appointment going forward in order to develop their new practice or research dimension. Those aiming for practice were given a 20% reduction for the fall semester to find and secure a practice. None needed this time; all who agreed to develop a practice were reappointed, and all had a practice contract before the end of the fall semester. I added the practice resources for that semester to their regular subsidized paychecks.

Researchers were given a 20% subsidy for 2 years. Even then, it was not enough time for junior or senior faculty unused to research productivity to get projects funded. A few stars made it within the time frame, but most needed a third year or left the faculty as they became frustrated with developing new competitive skills.

3
•••••

Developing the Three Dimensions
of Professional Contributions
•••••

IN THE RADICAL FIRST YEAR in our renewal, the faculty agreed to establish an innovative BS program for college graduates, devote time and effort to build a research presence, participate in a new and imaginative practice plan, and double their productivity.

The problems in the school were far broader, however, than ways in which faculty functioned. In a survey of the existing support staff and infrastructure in early 1986, the chair of that committee reported that staff were "grumbling and complaining that union involvement is strong. Much time is wasted writing and typing up unimportant incidents 'for the record.' At times, the atmosphere is extremely unprofessional in the (staff) area; occasional yelling, boisterous conversation, rowdy laughter, aimless walking around and disregard of the nonsmoking directive." A great number of faculty noted that "the secretary spends most of her time making and receiving personal phone calls." The report noted that the administrator in charge of support staff was "rude" and employed "destructive and unprofessional behavior" toward faculty. Faculty reported that secretaries have answered phone calls for them with comments that range from "she's in the bathroom" to "I have no idea where she is." Callback information was often lacking entirely or filled with inaccurate names or phone numbers. Clearly, support for faculty was in disarray.

We took a multidimensional approach to solving the many problems in the school: the eroding quality and number of student applicants, a diminished and single-focus faculty (teaching), assets being swallowed up by lack of productivity, and a university that fully expected the school to be extinguished or revert to its hospital roots. We had a lot to do in a short time, and with a looming catastrophe we felt free to innovate on a scale that a well-grounded and successful faculty would never have allowed.

The five committees that took shape within the first few weeks of my taking the dean position (I never used my formal title, "acting dean," because it denoted an impermanence that was not appropriate to the revolutionary part I wished to take) were meant to solve problems, but also to provide balance.

Committee 1

Teaching was the school's only strong point, but our approach was outdated. Four-year baccalaureate programs were losing ground, and we believed we needed to take a lead in developing a nursing program for college graduates. This kind of program belonged in a first-rate university like Columbia, but it was especially important for our school. Our school was located on the medical center campus 50 blocks north of the main campus and it included four health sciences schools, with nursing the only one with an undergraduate program. This distinguished us in a way that hampered our full partnership in the medical center as a health professions school. If we could transition our first degree in nursing to a graduate program, we would be taking a giant step to joining our medical center peers in educating only graduate students. Establishing a doctoral program was a longer-term goal, but transitioning our BS degree to a degree for college graduates was something we could do quickly.

Committee 2

In the same education arena, a faculty committee recommended ways to strengthen and consolidate our advanced practice MS programs. It was in these programs that we distinguished ourselves the most: We had the oldest midwifery MS program and pediatric nurse practitioners (NP) program in the country. We had too many small subspecialties, however. This committee strove to strengthen the MS programs, including introducing new courses in genetics and informatics—the first school to do so.

In an effort to respond to those advocates of the school who believed we must have closer alliances with the hospital, we tried to initiate programs that would do so but that would foster the independent functions of nursing: a new program for BS completion by nurses without the degree, and a clinical precepting program whereby hospital nurses gained status as formal preceptors of our students.

Committee 3

The most contentious committee was the committee on faculty practice. At Bendixen's demand, Dean Jamann had instituted a faculty practice task force in early 1985. The committee met monthly, and the minutes record an ongoing genda of information gathering from published articles, as well as debate over their responsibilities. At the May 12, 1985, meeting it was decided that their mission was to "serve as a reaction group for Health Sciences Administration development of clinical preceptorships." The committee missed the mark entirely and defaulted to medical center direction.

Seven months later, at the last task force meeting, the group planned to collect data on where faculty and students were adding clinical productivity as part of the education process.

The school was spinning out of control, relying on committees such as this one that could neither move in any forward direction nor take stock of why they should do so.

As we began renewed work in faculty practice in 1996, we determined to define it and differentiate it from research. The entire faculty voted by secret ballot on the committee's recommendation to require each faculty member to be engaged in research or in practice as a percentage of their full-time appointment. The result was nearly three to one in favor of the recommendation. The seven who rejected these new faculty-approved requirements resigned or their contracts for employment were not renewed.

Committee 4

MS programs were combined, strengthened, or eliminated, a new accelerated master's program (AMP) was developed for registered nurses (RNs) to obtain a BS and MS in a seamless and sequential program, and a new Entry to Practice (ETP) program was developed for college graduates to obtain a BS in nursing. By developing AMP and ETP, we opted out of the traditional BS degree programs; with all ETPs already college graduates and with AMP students enrolled in a seamless BS/MS degree, we built the bridge to an all-graduate degree school. Because ETP students earned a second BS degree with us, it was arguably about being an all-graduate-degree school, but ETPs were like medical, public health (PH), and dentistry students—post-baccalaureate students.

Committee 5

The fifth faculty committee designed a preceptorship program, which was aimed at enriching the clinical experience for students and assisting hospitals in recruiting our graduates. Students would be placed in one "host" hospital for all their clinical experience, and the hospital would assign their qualified staff as nurse preceptors with a highly intensive one on one assignment for the last semester. We invited five hospitals to participate (Presbyterian, Lenox Hill, Roosevelt, Memorial Sloan-Kettering Cancer Center, and Mt. Sinai). All but Presbyterian joined in the partnership.

Faculty practice was preferentially established at the partnership hospitals. The partnership hospitals' nurse credentials, salary, and fringe rates were similar to those of Columbia School of Nursing, so reimbursement for faculty practice presented no problems. However, Presbyterian Hospital had different resources and benefits. Their salary fringe rate at the time was 17% versus 27% at Columbia; Presbyterian declined to provide the additional 10% needed for faculty salary benefits. Presbyterian alone among our proposed partnership hospitals required all nurses to join the union, including those in faculty practice. When these issues were determined by the university to be unacceptable, the hospital proposed, instead, a "reverse" faculty practice whereby Presbyterian hospital would "sell" time of their staff to teach rather than hire Columbia faculty to practice. When we declined to participate in this model (the hospital had very few RN staff who met educational qualifications for a faculty position), the hospital offered to hire faculty as part-time staff with no fringe benefits. These were very frustrating issues for us as we tried to sustain Presbyterian as our premier partner. The hospital nursing structure was too disparate from other New York City medical center hospitals, making a partnership with us very difficult.

While our school was moving rapidly in the spring of 1986 to redesign faculty roles and student experiences, Presbyterian was still making plans according to their January expectations that Presbyterian would become the clinical determinant of the school's survival, and receive recognition by overseeing and renaming the school. In early 1986, faculty and administrative offices were split between two buildings: the administrative building of the medical school and the Georgian Building. Mismatched and decrepit furniture was moved into rooms that had been dorm spaces in the Georgian, and little was done to paint or repair floors. Memorabilia, art, silver, grandfather clocks, and furniture from Maxwell Hall had been distributed among offices at Presbyterian Hospital (or the home of one of its former executives) since they believed Maxwell Hall and its historical treasure was their initial and current property. The school had intellectually morphed to the university but not its accommodations or belongings. Later in the year, Presbyterian Hospital president Thomas Morris gave us access to some remaining portraits and engraved bowls, and allowed us to have one of the original grandfather clocks from Maxwell Hall installed in the Georgian Building lobby. He admonished me to take good care of it. The vice president of nursing said to me 4 months into my deanship "you are a moving target; we can't understand how to work with you." That same month, in a letter dated April 24, 1986, she wrote me proposing that the future of nursing excellence at the medical center "demands that individually held resources are utilized jointly." The proposal was eerily reminiscent of Tom Morris's letter of December 1985 when I was appointed. A new model of clinical education for Columbia students was again proposed in the April 1986 letter whereby all Columbia students would be educated at Presbyterian and Presbyterian nurses would be the sole clinical instructors. Students would work 32 hours a week at the hospital, receive a stipend for half of those hours, and their "student clinical experience will be distributed over seven days of the week with patterns of classes scheduled to provide an interface." This model could have come directly out of the 1892 founding design of the school. Nearly 100 years later, it was resurfacing. The hospital recommended that "recognition be given to the unique contribution of the Division of Nursing at Presbyterian by modifying the name of the school to include the hospital name" in the some form. Example: "Columbia Presbyterian School of Nursing." They further stated that "the clinical program model will be the property of Presbyterian . . . and may be marketed to other BS schools of nursing in the future."

The dissonance between Columbia Nursing and Presbyterian, and the school's struggle to catch up with academic nursing expectations, caused a division of purpose that still exists. Compounding the dissonance was the

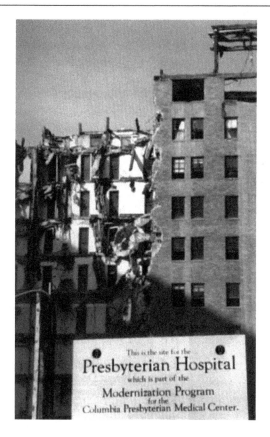

Maxwell Hall's last days in 1984.

● ● ● ● ●

presence of a 2-year associate degree nursing program within Presbyterian (The Clark School) and the distant and unusual functioning of an alumni association, which was largely led by nurses who had stayed at Presbyterian following graduation and who wished to sustain the hospital base for the school. All of these factors played a part in the troubled relationship of the hospital and school.

By the end of the first semester, our first successes were already apparent in the area of research: five new doctorally prepared faculty had been recruited, two of whom brought research grants with them. Five senior administrative positions had been filled, and plans were made to address a budget that had one third of its revenues going toward common costs for the university, a higher percentage than that of any of the other 15 schools at Columbia. The physical deterioration of the school's space was documented in 35 photographs submitted to the university. Emerging successes had given way to new challenges.

The provost, Dr. Goldberger, advised me that he would not begin the formal search for a dean unless a formal review of the school was first conducted. Therefore, on September 11, 1986, he commissioned an internal review committee of three physicians, two nurses, and seven university staff. In this letter to the committee, he wrote, in part:

> In professional opportunities for women, the changing role of the nursing professional in our society, the high cost of tuition and college, and changes in the nursing school program have all contributed to an instability in enrollment and faculty. Thus, we must seriously consider the current status of the school and must plan for the future.
>
> Among the options you should consider are:
>
> a. Following Dr. Mundinger's plan now under development (which did not depend on a unification with Presbyterian) or
> b. Devising a new program involving closer ties with Presbyterian; and incorporating some components of the school program into other parts of the Health Sciences Division (such as the School of Public Health) while phasing out other components (such as the BS program).
>
> You should report to me no later than December 1986.

The committee, deeply divided and contentious in its deliberations, did not meet the Goldberger deadline.

The review of the school committee rolled past its December 1986 report deadline, and the committee did not finish its work until 9 months later, in October 1987, and even then, there were two reports, not one: a "majority report" signed by six committee members and a "minority report" signed by four committee members. During those months, the nursing faculty continued their brave and productive work strengthening a school they hoped the university would sustain. Bendixen, the center of the school's support, was advised by President Sovern in June of 1987 that a search for Bendixen's replacement would begin immediately, a step the medical school faculty successfully reversed in a strong plea to the president. Weeks later the president himself took a year's leave of absence, and Provost Goldberger became acting president—a position he held when the nursing review report was finally submitted.

Fate had once again intervened in our favor. The plan had been clear: The provost would commission a report, he would review the independent assessment of the state of the school, and he would act on it. This approach was academically sound and above reproach, but we knew he had made up his mind guided by the individuals he had named to the committee, which included only two nurses out of a committee of 10. But as he awaited the overdue but expected report from those he had handpicked to reflect his views, he was whisked away to a higher station—acting president—at the very time the report was wending its way to the provost's office. Fortunately for us, he wasn't there to receive it. And happily for us, Goldberger could move to his new office as acting president. And thankfully for the "rebels" in the committee, the report had been delayed for months as the chair unsuccessfully attempted to bring order and consensus to her deeply divided commission.

A minority report issued by just less than half the committee focused on the successes already apparent and the promise of continued survival. The majority report, however, saw things differently. Their summation from the associate provost, Kathleen Mullinix, who chaired the committee concluded:

A leadership position would be achieved if Columbia's School of Nursing would distinguish itself from others by focusing on education and patient care. There is no requirement for the development of a tenured, research oriented faculty or for the granting of a research degree.

Even with its recommendations for the school to return to its hospital-based clinical roots, the majority report ended with a paragraph stating many on the committee had "serious doubt" that a large number of people would be willing to pay tuition for a nursing education in the private sector that was very high relative to their expected income, and to assume a role that had come to be considered, for a variety of unfortunate reasons, menial.

Bendixen sent a blistering response to Mullinix regarding the report, listing 19 inaccurate or baldly biased sections. Some of his comments were acidly humorous, as when he responded to the quote in the report: "A majority of the members could not define a body of knowledge and experience that is substantive and unique to nursing." He responded that "since only two of the 12 members of the task force were nurses, this is not surprising."

In commenting on the fact that the committee sought only one external consultant—a nurse administrator without a doctorate—he rebutted the committee observation that research was not necessary in a school of nursing: "This suggests the unrealistic expectation that care can be divorced from research. One cannot expect nursing care to be taught in the absence of teachers who are engaged in advancing the knowledge base of that care; certainly not when excellence is the goal." He cited several quotes from reports or interviews that were 180 degrees from what the record showed had transpired, calling into question not just the sloppiness and bias of the report, but the honesty of those who wrote it. His letter was met with total silence from the provost's office. The report served to energize the faculty, whose respect for their profession had been brutally challenged by this assessment. Instead of a death knell, these words fueled a response of indignation and renewed commitment.

In 1987, with President Sovern on leave and Provost Goldberger serving as acting president, the report to the provost fell into the hands of Fritz Stern, a distinguished professor of history who had once earlier in his career served as acting provost and now once again had been appointed to this interim role. Wise, seasoned, and a brilliant scholar, Stern had no biases about nursing. While Goldberger had immediately gone to the National Institutes of Health (NIH) directly out of his residency training—never experiencing the nuances of clinical care and the contributions of academic nursing—Stern simply knew us as one of 16 schools at Columbia and when he took a look he liked what he saw. So the report to Provost Stern was read with amusement and skepticism, spurred no response, and was simply filed as a part of those turbulent years. My plan went forward. Without this cascade of changing responsibilities—Sovern on leave, Goldberger in the president's office, and Stern in the provost position—our fate might have been different.

The end-of-year annual report in 1987, 2 years after I became dean, describes new federal funding obtained during the year for three MS programs, 21 faculty practice contracts in place, a new clinical program proposed at Presbyterian Hospital whereby a unit staffed by nursing faculty would be established for teaching purposes, the announcement that the *Journal of Professional Nursing* (the journal of the American Association of Colleges of Nursing) was devoting an entire issue to the Columbia Nursing innovations, increased federal aid related to success in recruiting minority students, and the development of a polished recruitment plan. Not only had revenues doubled, but the school had spent only $3 million of its $4 million revenues, providing a transfer to the endowment of $1 million. We were beginning to raise real money from alumni and corporations for our endowment, especially from those who saw our new ideas worthy of funding. With growth in the university endowment, ours now reached $6 million, or five times what we had after paying off our debts in 1986.

In March 1988, Goldberger, back in his provost office, agreed that the school could go forward, with an understanding that the school would close its BS program and send more students to Presbyterian. These goals were somewhat conflicting since the hospital could not provide clinical experiences for MS-level students.

THE SEARCH FOR A PERMANENT DEAN

The search committee for a permanent dean of nursing was announced on March 3. In April, the chair of the search committee, Lewis Rowland (chair of Neurology), called to discuss the process with me. He asked if I'd be a candidate and I responded, "yes" —but only with a decision on my candidacy reached by the committee before looking externally for candidates or advertising the search. I was having fun and wanted to support the faculty in the new and exciting turnaround. I said my early success and path that I had charted was what the university wanted, or they should decide now to look elsewhere. I said if candidates were sought or public announcement of a search were made, I would resign immediately.

While the committee pondered their moves, the faculty continued its efforts with Presbyterian, mostly enhanced clinical education opportunities and renewed efforts with faculty practices. Since Presbyterian nursing did not have positions for advanced practice clinicians, as all other New York City hospitals had, it was difficult to develop faculty practice or clinical education for our master's students. Presbyterian administrators tried to work with us to find common purpose, but a proposed teaching unit—with faculty paid by the hospital to staff an inpatient unit and include students—could not be fully staffed because of the disparity between hospital and school salaries.

At the same time, we struggled with inadequate security near our space in the Georgian Building (several student muggings and thefts had occurred) and a continued physical deterioration in the building. We had won an academic reprieve but not a physical one; our building was a disaster. In March 1988, the National League for Nursing (NLN) conducted its 10-year review of the school and recommended that a new, better space was required. On June 16, the deputy vice president for Health Sciences facilities, Lou Saksen, advised me that a triangle of land a block away from us was potentially available for a new School of Nursing building. He estimated the total cost of the building would be $2.5 million; we figured we could pay for it outright from our endowment. As medical center space planning went forward that year, this opportunity disappeared.

Although Goldberger had asked that the school close its BS program, the medical school faculty (under Bendixen's urging) filed a faculty resolution with the provost that the BS program should continue (in its new format for college graduates) and that it served our collaborative efforts with PH; Goldberger never responded. That fall we accepted our first class of extremely promising new students—34 in total—into the ETP program.

In July, after 4 months of meetings (no ads, no search), the committee recommended me as dean to Provost Goldberger. He phoned me to offer me the position, and as I asked him the parameters of the appointment, he told me the appointment did not come with tenure, since that had not explicitly been included in his charge to the committee and that, furthermore, he did not believe it was merited. I told him that tenure was a requirement for me, and I therefore declined his offer of appointment. Since the school had no tenured faculty, I believed it would be difficult indeed to build a tenured faculty if the dean were untenured. That evening President Sovern called me at home and said he wanted me to accept the appointment, with tenure, and said "the door was open" for the development of the doctoral program. I accepted.

FINANCIAL CHALLENGES AND FINANCIAL GAINS

In 1988, the Alumni Association endowment remained at $4 million, including $48,000 in new revenues for the year (dues and gifts). Only minimal funding to the school was forthcoming, but scholarships were awarded to Columbia alumni to attend other schools, notably New York University where several alumni officers were employed. The fissure between the association and the school was growing deeper. Faculty salaries were up 50% from 1985, and student enrollments had risen to 234 from 178 in 1985; the difference of our full-time equivalents (FTEs) was even more stunning: 201 in 1988 in comparison to 65 in 1985. This was primarily due to required full-time enrollment in the new ETP program. Two federal research awards were granted to faculty, including the first-ever NIH grant awarded to a Columbia University School of Nursing (CUSN) researcher, Joyce Anastasi.

UNIVERSITY COST ASSESSMENT TO THE SCHOOL OF NURSING

The year 1989 marked the appointment of Herbert Pardes as the new vice president for Health Sciences. He had previously been chair of psychiatry, and his political skills were superb. Pardes negotiated stunningly new financial relationships between the health sciences and the central university, which helped health sciences develop a strong and separate four-school entity and have a more transparent and lower health science assessment for university common costs. For the first time, all indirect costs recovered from NIH grants would come in full to the schools in the medical center where they were awarded instead of being targeted at 80% by the central university. As these new algorithms were developed, I argued in a February 7, 1989, memo that common costs attributed to the School of Nursing should be far less than they had been. I noted that

- Only 72 of our 426 students, unlike medicine and dentistry, were full time and that using head count as a proxy for service utilizations was too high.
- With an average student age of 30, most lived off campus and did not use the same proportion of services as the other health sciences students who lived on campus.

- Of 894 health sciences students residing on campus only 29 (3%) were nursing students.
- Only 10% of our students were assigned for clinical practice in the medical center, again supporting less use of services.
- Library use by "nurses" included three times as many hospital nurses and The Clark School students as were in the Columbia School of Nursing, therefore substantiating a reduction in our assigned costs for the library.
- Space allocations were also overstated for the School of Nursing, and an argument was made that quality (as well as quantity) of space and priority for classroom space (which influenced assignment of optimum classrooms) should be a factor in cost allocation.

Although steeped in good data, nothing came of our pleas. Common costs for the medical center were a zero-sum game; any reduction of cost for us would mean a corresponding increase for another health sciences school. The fact that we had more surplus resources than any other school also eroded our argument about being overcharged. In fact, in 1989—for the first time—Columbia nursing salaries exceeded the national average for schools of nursing's located in academic health centers.

IMPROVING FINANCIALS AND ESTABLISHING A BUILDING FUND

Research was funded from five private foundations (Kellogg, Pfizer, Rudin, American Cancer Society, and Diamond) for nearly $2 million. These funds paid for research faculty salaries, allowing a school surplus of $1.1 million to be transferred to the endowment. Enrollments were up 40% from the low of 1985. Sources of nontuition revenues in 1989 were four times what they were in 1985 ($3,351,651 from $800,588). In one way our frugality, new productivity, and investment planning worked against us. Whereas many other schools in the university were struggling to support their (sometimes bloated) endeavors, we had pared down our expenses to only what we needed and could afford, making us appear flush with resources. Schools whose missions had long been revered by the university were more likely to be propped up financially than a school like ours, which had appeared so recently to be unsalvageable. If we were to survive, we would be doing it on our own, and paradoxically, the better we did, the less likely we would receive help. After all, there were so many other schools far more in need than ours.

A new building fund was established with $400,000 in school funds available because revenues from hospitals supplemented our financial aid budget. The partnerships we established with five hospitals included agreements with students to practice in those hospitals after graduation in return for financial aid. This freed up school money for a building fund. The fund established in 1989 was unique in the university that year because of the general state of university finances. For example, the medical school budget showed that $158,000 had been spent from the capital in its endowment, and the School of Public Health budget eroded its endowment by $23,000. That year, total debits from school endowments totaled $6 million; at the same time, the nursing school showed a surplus of nearly 25% of revenues, all of which was added to the endowment. A letter to deans and vice presidents from the provost outlined the university's conservative expectations for 1989 capital spending, including specific guidance regarding new buildings.

"Given the conditions of our buildings, the limited availability of suitable building sites in this area, and the cost of new constructions . . . most projects will be on the refurbishment of existing buildings." He went on to say that 5-year plans for building construction "should be of sufficient priority that strong consideration would be given to fund raising or debt financing for them in lieu of other pressing operating needs such as financial aid and faculty salaries."

No longer feeling the threat of insolvency in the School of Nursing, we had many priorities for our growing assets. Financial aid had quadrupled with our new program. From a school based primarily on self-pay part-time students, we were becoming a school primarily focused on full-time students, who were increasingly eligible for financial aid. We had also raised faculty salaries significantly, competing with the rising salaries in practice, as all professional schools must do (law, medicine, business), but also placing nursing faculty salaries in the higher levels of all Columbia faculty. We had worked hard to fund the salaries and financial aid, and now the most critical need was a new building. Provost Goldberger's letter opened the door for this possibility in his letter suggesting, "debt financing" for a building. That we could do. Our investments in the endowment were growing fast enough to yield sufficient income to pay off the debt we would need to build a new building. We believed the best use of our assets was to continue investing every saved and earned dollar into the endowment, with a focus on a new building.

4

•••••

Anchoring Our Endeavor

•••••

NOTWITHSTANDING THE CONFLICTING VIEW ON the nature and contributions of a nursing school to the university, Provost Goldberger was always ultimately supportive of my requests and approved, and even offered, resources for our success. Although his approval in 1988 for the continuation of the school included a plan to close the baccalaureate program, he nonetheless acceded the next year to a reformulation of the BS degree program, which would be the initial degree for college graduates pursuing the combined BS and advanced practice MS degree (our Entry to Practice [ETP] program), and he assisted us with New York State approvals. In the same 1988 agreement, he asked that any tuition we raised over the current enrollment numbers would be utilized in very restrictive ways, but by spring 1989 he was willing to approve my plan for broader investments in the future and even exempted them from the conventional tax to the central university. Similarly, he approved our plan to begin to develop a doctoral program in 1989, although he had opposed this plan during his review of the school. Goldberger also agreed to consider reduction of our common cost assessment. When I was appointed dean in 1988, I was also appointed—by Goldberger—to the university Budget and Planning Committee. Experience on the committee gave me substantive education about university financing, budgeting, and overall economic strategy. It was crucial to my restructuring of nursing's financial contributions and benefits in the following years. Most importantly, he came to understand and support our financial and professional independence in regard to joint efforts with the Presbyterian Hospital. All of these approvals, exemptions, and understandings with Provost Goldberger were critical to our emerging renewal.

During these first 5 years, the new plan for precepting with four of our major hospital affiliates grew, and faculty practice was thriving. The only painfully missing partner was Presbyterian Hospital, which declined to participate in the precepting program. In addition, faculty practice at

Presbyterian Hospital was marginal, because of limited positions for advanced practice and benefits that were not in line with Columbia's. Presbyterian Hospital president and the vice president for nursing wanted to join us in stronger partnerships, but the structure, history, resources, and expectations of the two nursing entities were far apart. Columbia was focused on advanced practice and hoped to develop the same par relationship that existed between university physicians who were trained and practiced at the hospital. In comparison, Presbyterian Hospital sustained a unionized workforce without an advanced practice component.

The ETP program established during these years proved to be an enormous benefit to nursing's growing professional recognition. The students were academically gifted (their SATs were within 4% of Columbia College's entering class), but what was most important they brought a maturity to their decision to become nurses. At the average age of 34, they had significant career and work experience, and carried no bias about the role of nursing in society. Although traditional nursing students entering nursing education fresh out of high school may have been equally qualified, determined, and attuned, their age and lack of prior college experience worked against them. Other professions—medicine, law, dentistry—were graduate endeavors, adding gravitas and importance. With the advent of entry-level education for college graduates, nursing took a major leap forward; the content of the education might not look that different from conventional nursing education but the new students did.

While path-finding achievements in faculty practice and educational innovations were established, our financial success was outpacing the university's and provided a new perspective on how the school underwrote its endeavors. During our first 5 years of renewal, the university encountered financial deficits in nearly every school and centrally. The late 1980s were difficult years. Perhaps because our school was not threatened, our attention was riveted early on solutions—and we were better able to withstand the downturn. Through faculty practice, we subsidized 20% of faculty salaries; from 1989 to 1991, we were the only Columbia school to award faculty salary percentage increases at the maximum allowed by the university. Indeed, some years we received approval to exceed that maximum level because of our resources. We not only benefited from faculty practice funds, but our total revenue increased more than fourfold during these 5 years, from $800,588 to $3,351,651. And each dollar over our penurious expenditures went to the endowment, which by the end of our first 5 years was $7.5 million, compared with our post-debt endowment of $1 million in 1985.

While the practice and educational models were extremely innovative, we sought to develop a strong—but conventional—nursing research program. We believed research by nurse scholars was proving to be a necessary "third leg" of academic success. Without it, there would be no rigorous testing of our new ideas, no new themes to measure, no platform in which to highlight nursing's accomplishments. As our sophisticated model grew, it was far more than two separate entities, but began to weave together the fabric of a school that valued its fundamental contribution to society—care for individuals—while teaching students how to learn ever-changing and improving nursing care, and how to measure those accomplishments.

President Sovern asked the right questions, and while keeping his distance, always gave me his support, but it was the next vice president for Health Sciences, Herbert Pardes, who provided not only the support but the context within which the school could solidify its gains and move into a position of credible leadership. In his 10 years as vice president for Health Sciences, Pardes never once declined my request for assistance. He was responsible for the long awaited full-school status for us, helped me recruit faculty who could secure tenure, and supported the establishment of our first endowed chair. Pardes negotiated independence for the health sciences schools, and then built a powerhouse of intellectual and vibrantly engaged faculty and a richly endowed enterprise. This was fertile ground and perfect timing for nursing's fledgling renewal to take root and flourish.

In the first 5 years, four influential physicians, in nonclinical roles, made it possible for the school to survive. Vice President for Health Sciences Bendixen and Trustee Hubbard were guardians at the gate, protecting me until our fledgling ideas took hold; another was Provost Goldberger, who played the role of judge, jury, and modest advocate within the university; and the fourth was Dr. Pardes, the new vice president for Health Sciences, who gave us full rein, confidence, and active support to chart our successful and promising future in the medical center. These were tumultuous times, for the challenge required nursing to provide enormous effort, gifted faculty and administrators, innovative programs, and money. All this was accomplished, and it was not the only time that a Columbia physician made the difference by putting his own eminence on the line for our untested ideas; this would happen again 8 years later, again with happy results.

Section II

• • • • •

The Medicaid Experiment:
1990–1995

• • • • •

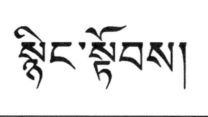

5

•••••

Primary Care Shortage

•••••

ALTHOUGH THERE HAVE BEEN DECADES of attempts to encourage physicians to become primary care doctors, few have been attracted to the role. Even fewer took that path in the 1990s, opening up opportunities in nursing. Many of the attempts to attract physicians into primary care included reimbursement enhancement (never enough) or models like team practice or medical home, where essentially the primary care physician is the leader and nurse practitioners give the care. The fundamental reasons physicians don't like primary care are not amenable to these attempts. Primary care doesn't pay nearly as well as specialty medicine; it doesn't have the same prestige, the hours are worse, and the content is mostly chronic illness care. Chronic illness care has challenges, for sure, but the competence needed in chronic care management transcends the scope of diagnostic and treatment modalities that draw individuals into a medical career. Nursing, however, has found primary care (and chronic illness care) to be a very satisfying specialty; keeping people well, avoiding the consequences of poor control of illness, developing social support, diagnosing illness, and giving care—all these are part of nursing's specialties.

Physicians in medical centers often provide primary care, but usually this care is given within their specialty. Cardiologists, neurologists, and others manage patients with chronic disease. Few medical center physicians, however, devote themselves to bread-and-butter primary care. Even though physicians are not attracted to primary care, conventional medical groups have been dead set against nurse practitioners having independent authority for this specialty; the biggest reason appears to be that this would acknowledge nurses as peers in primary care, a bridge many physicians have no intention of crossing.

Medical center physicians are different in this regard. Most are specialists, and they deeply value primary care colleagues who can make knowledgeable referrals for specialty care and who can assume qualified primary care referrals from specialists.

There is one exception to this: anesthesiologists. This specialty probably has the closest overlap of any area of medicine where nurses and physicians practice, making the exquisitely defined differences inflamed areas of contention. In many sites, anesthesiologists may "supervise" as many as four nurse anesthetists at any given time, and are richly paid to do so. This may be what some physicians in primary care hope to emulate in order to designate certain tasks to nurse practitioners (NPs) in their practices, and keep the more interesting and complex encounters for themselves, but for them the opportunity has passed. Nurse practitioners already have been accepted as primary care providers in every state, some independently and some in a variety of medical doctor collaborations, but the confining regulations are disappearing as the need for primary care grows and the quality of NP care is better recognized. Regardless of the hundreds of published articles attesting to the high quality of NP care, the tipping point for full acknowledgment of NPs had not yet been reached in 1990. Skeptics pointed to data that showing NPs could perform only 70% to 85% of what a primary care physician could do, and they took more time doing it. No comparison studies had yet been done where NPs had the same authority and patient population as medical doctors: If NPs didn't have full prescriptive authority, or hospital or emergency room (ER) privileges, or the access and ability to order and analyze imaging studies, then of course they couldn't measure up to 100% of the medical doctor scope of care. It wasn't a nurse deficit; it was a regulatory deficit. Do nurses really take more time giving care? Maybe yes and maybe no. Because nurses incorporate more teaching, for both patients and families, are more likely to seek community services to support patients' recovery, and are more likely to use an acute illness encounter to address broader health issues, they will take more time. In practices where a physician and NP may share a panel of patients, it is much more likely for the NP to be caring far more chronically ill patients, who are the most time-consuming practice components. But with patient encounters where the process and content of care is the same, there is no evidence that nurses are slower.

In the mid-1990s, a document was developed for Columbia physicians who were establishing the Columbia Physicians Provider Network (CPPN). The purpose of the document was to lay out the pros and cons of the Columbia network contracting with health maintenance organizations (HMOs) and preferred provider organizations (PPOs). One of the most serious concerns was that the CPPN did not have an adequate number of primary care physicians to make referrals to Columbia physician specialists within any given network. They feared that if they joined HMO/PPO networks they might be cut out of a significant number of referrals. The CPPN had been established to deal with the expected increasing presence of managed care organizations, and they saw that primary care was a fundamental asset in the new and emerging HMO market. Columbia physicians were acutely aware of this missing asset in proposed network contracts. Fear about overlap between the professions is of little concern to physicians well grounded in their specialties. Our faculty practice model, just 4 years old, was almost exclusively in primary care sites: pediatrics, family practice, and adult primary care. The faculty nurse practitioners' academic standing had already given them unique recognition in the medical center. They stood out not only for their excellence in care, but also as professors who taught students, participated in scientific studies led by research faculty, and published articles about their clinical work. Revenues from faculty practices subsidized the salaries of these clinicians. This was the National Institutes of Health (NIH) analogue for clinicians. It was in this environment that new primary care efforts became established in our school.

In 1993, our researchers, a small and distinguished group, were beginning to obtain federal funding for their work, from both the NIH and private health foundations. We recruited Kristine Gebbie, who was the founding national director for President Clinton's AIDS organization and had been the state director of health in both Washington and Oregon. Gebbie was enormously successful as an academic and grounded our public health presence. Joyce Anastasi, our first NIH-funded scholar, continued with prodigious productivity in AIDS research and became a magnet for recruiting students and faculty. Mary Byrne, Carol Roye, Dick Garfield, and Donna Gaffney were innovative and well-regarded researchers, even this early in their careers. The high-profile Entry to Practice program was attracting well-qualified applicants at a time when many college graduates were struggling to find rewarding careers. Our research—practice—education plan had begun to bear fruit, not only in building our future in each area, but in building the connections among the three, which would ultimately be the design for our academic presence.

6

•••••

Luck Comes to Those Who Prepare for It

•••••

OUR FACULTY PRACTICE TOOK A new and exciting path in 1993. New York City medical centers were consolidating by buying smaller independent hospitals, and most were also investing millions in new facilities. William Speck, MD, the Presbyterian Hospital president and CEO, was part of the New York City–wide expansion, but he had a unique challenge. With Presbyterian Hospital's enterprise, which included Harlem Hospital, and located within a low-income neighborhood in northwest Manhattan, the demand for services (especially from underserved, low-paying Medicaid patients) was higher than in many other New York City medical center areas. Cornell's New York Hospital and Mt. Sinai on the east side, and New York University in a mostly upscale lower eastside location, had less demand, proportionately, from underserved populations. Therefore, when Presbyterian sought low-interest funding for its new mainframe from New York State, the approval came with strings attached.

In order to access the preferred loan, Presbyterian would be required to increase primary care services for underserved populations who lived near the hospital. Speck, who had run Rainbow Hospital for Children in Philadelphia at the University of Pennsylvania, had a pediatrician's heart as well as a gifted administrator's brain. He believed deeply in helping poor families and readily agreed to the New York State proposal. His initial effort, most naturally, was to seek support for primary care development from Columbia's medical school faculty. Although Herb Pardes was ideologically supportive and believed in the same goals as Bill Speck, the primary care resources in the Columbia's medical school looked like primary resources in most prestigious medical centers: sparse and were already overwhelmed. Primary care as a necessary part of internal medicine and pediatrics was alive and well, but no excess resources existed to increase availability of services to the underserved population.

By the summer of 1993, all clinical nursing faculty had practices, many with physicians at Presbyterian Hospital and its community hospital, Allen Pavilion. Therefore, it was not surprising that the second part of Bill Speck's search for primary care clinicians found us. Would we be willing to partner with Presbyterian by staffing two new primary care practices?

Because faculty already had established satisfying practices, many would be reluctant to relinquish them to join this initiative. It would be important to enrich the new opportunity to attract their participation. We also hoped to take this unique opportunity to evaluate a nurse-run practice from the very first day of development. In order to do this, I proposed that we seek funding for an evaluation of the new practice, comparing it to physicians practicing in sites and with patients comparable to ours. Speck readily agreed, but we both knew that primary care nurses in existing nursing practice held less authority than their physician counterparts. This meant that comparability would be difficult to measure. Physicians had hospital admitting privileges and potentially influential cross-site management that could bias a comparability study. In the first meeting with me in the spring of 1993 when Speck introduced the idea of nurse-run practices, I asked if he would agree to hospital admitting/management responsibilities for faculty nurse practitioners in the new practices so that we could conduct the first reliable comparability study. He immediately said yes, and so it was that a landmark study and nurse independence had their genesis. All we had to do was find a way to operationalize this new authority.

The new practice would require new knowledge as well as new authority, and there was only one route to get there—through the Department of Medicine. Mike Weisfeldt, chair of medicine, immediately and enthusiastically gave us support and the means to develop this new initiative.

During the summer and fall, with the full support of Pardes and Weisfeldt, a plan was formalized to grant admitting privileges to faculty nurse practitioners (NPs). New York State already allowed NPs to independently prescribe all drugs, and also authorized independent practice with a written MD collaborative agreement. (This agreement essentially guaranteed MD counsel when sought by the NP, but no practice oversight or supervision was required.) The state, however, required an MD signature within 24 hours of any hospital admission, and we would have to build this requirement into our new plan.

Medicaid, which would be the major payer for these newly served patients, benefited from this project in many ways. State by state, Medicaid policy differed in payment given to NPs, ranging from 50% to 100% of the physician fee schedule in each state. In New York State, Medicaid paid 100% of the MD fee schedule to NPs. This gave us fee comparability, which would make it easier to distinguish cost of care differences between MDs and NPs. Freestanding primary care practice for Medicaid patients was not sustainable under fees then paid by New York State, but these new proposed practices carried an enhanced reimbursement fee schedule because they were within a hospital system, an important New York State waiver for hospitals, with primary care clinics. We therefore had comparable, and sufficient, revenues with which to conduct the new practices.

In December 1993, the Medical Board passed a resolution to authorize admitting privileges for faculty NPs and midwives for the initial 2 years of our new practice. The new policy stated that the chief of the medical school, vice president of nursing at Presbyterian Hospital, and the dean of the nursing school would each sign the application of every nurse faculty clinician, and that only faculty from the nursing school were eligible for such an appointment. The addition of the signature of the hospital's vice president for nursing helped assure that the NPs would have good relationships with hospital staff nurses on the units where NPs admitted patients.

THE ESTABLISHMENT OF THE CENTER FOR ADVANCED PRACTICE

Both medical center and university publications ran articles on this significant new policy. Bill Speck and I had agreed that faculty selected for the newly named Center for Advanced Practice (CAP) would relinquish their current practices April 1, to allow 6 months of additional training, fit out the new space, and other planning required. Speck had agreed to pay hospital salaries for the 6-month "residency" as well as the salaries for the ensuing practices, which would have Medicaid reimbursement accruing to the hospital. Eventually the date for the opening of the practice was delayed until December 1994. Midwives and pediatric NPs would be involved, as well as adult/family NPs. Midwifery admission privileges were to occur, Speck wrote, "as part of a corrective action plan" with New York State. The faculty midwives therefore were to be part of a state-funded improved obstetrical care program agreed to by Presbyterian.

In April, the medical board approved the specific policy and procedures for faculty NP admitting privileges (see p. 42). One by one the chairmen of all the departments voted yes: Bickers (Dermatology), Weisfeldt (Medicine), Fox (OB), Shelansky (Pathology), Driscoll (Pediatrics), Reemtsma (Surgery), Rowland (Neurology), Alderson (Radiology), Lieberman (Rehab), Stein (Neurosurgery), Rose (Surgery)—but last, with a high stack of documents in front of him to support his vote, Ed Miller, chairman of anesthesiology, voted no. I knew he would vote no; the long-inflamed relationship over the independence of nurse anesthetists made it likely Miller would follow the path his anesthesiologist colleagues and organization had long taken. After all, there was big money in the current system of paying anesthesiologists to "supervise" nurse anesthetists in the operating room—supervision that lacked substance, if one was to observe the process. Ed Miller left Columbia in late 1996 to become dean of the medical school and vice president for health sciences at Johns Hopkins University. He has served there with great distinction. Early in his tenure at Hopkins, he wrote me a long letter telling me his vote on admitting privileges for NPs had been based not on personal conviction, but on his professional role at the time.

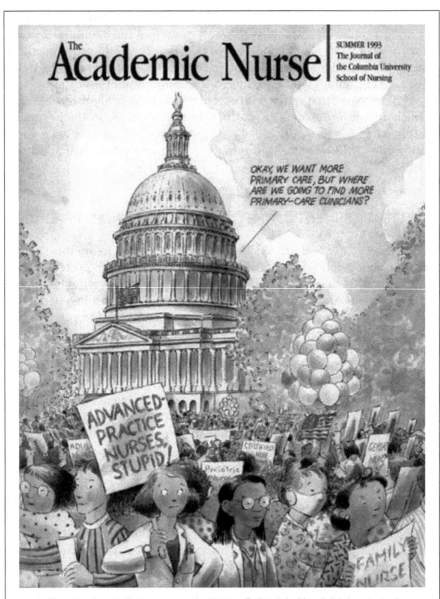

The Academic Nurse *cover depicting Columbia Nursing's pursuit of independent primary care by nurses.*

• • • • •

The Presbyterian Hospital
in the City of New York
Columbia - Presbyterian Medical Center
New York, NY 10032 - 3784

DATE ISSUED	NUMBER
ISSUED MAY 4, 1994	12.9402

APPROVED	PAGE
MEDICAL BOARD 4/20/94	1 OF 3

MEDICAL BOARD

POLICY AND PROCEDURE MANUAL

FACULTY NURSE PRACTITIONERS-ADMITTING PRIVILEGES

POLICY

Subject to the conditions stated below, nurse practitioners who are members of the full time Faculty of the Columbia University School of Nursing (hereinafter Faculty NP's) may be granted privileges to admit patients to the Medical, Pediatric of Obstetrics and Gynecology Services of The Presbyterian Hospital in the City of New York (the "Hospital").

CONDITIONS

1. A Faculty NP applying for admitting privileges must be credentialed to perform services at the Hospital pursuant to the Hospital's Special Health Nursing Professional Policy.

2. A Faculty NP applying for admitting privileges must be a member of the faculty of the Columbia University School of Nursing and be recommended by its Dean for such admitting privileges.

3. A Faculty NP applying for admitting privileges must be credentialed to perform all of the services necessary to carry out his or her responsibilities in connection with admitting privileges.

4. A Faculty NP applying for admitting privileges must have in effect a detailed written collaborative practice agreement with his or her attending physician and have the terms of such agreement approved in writing by the Director of the appropriate Service of the Hospital, which sets forth the terms upon which admitting privileges are conditioned, including how orders are written for patients, when consultations must be requested by the Faculty NP, and when and how patients will be transferred to other units of the Hospital. Each agreement shall provide that the physician's opinion shall prevail in any disagreements between the physician, or any covering physician, and the Faculty NP with regard to patient management.

PURPOSE

To permit Faculty NP's to admit patients to the Hospital, to assure that these individuals are properly qualified and have appropriate privileges.

The Allen Pavilion • Dana W. Atchley Pavilion • Babies Hospital • The Edward S. Harkness Eye Institute • Milstein Hospital Building
Harkness Pavilion • Neurological Institute • New York Orthopaedic Hospital • Sloane Hospital • Squier Urological Clinic • Vanderbilt Clinic

● ● ● ● ●

The Presbyterian Hospital
in the City of New York
Columbia - Presbyterian Medical Center
New York, NY 10032 - 3784

DATE ISSUED	NUMBER
ISSUED MAY 4, 1994	12.9402
APPROVED	PAGE
MEDICAL BOARD 4/20/94	2 OF 3

MEDICAL BOARD
POLICY AND PROCEDURE MANUAL

PURPOSE

To permit Faculty NP's to admit patients to the Hospital, to assure that these individuals are properly qualified and have appropriate privileges.

APPLICABILITY

This policy shall apply only to Faculty NP's who apply for and receive admitting privileges at The Presbyterian Hospital for the period ending with the 1995/96 academic year at which time this policy shall be reevaluated.

PROCEDURE

1. A Faculty NP applying for admitting privileges shall submit a written application for such privileges to the Hospital's Senior Vice President for Medical Affairs. Such request shall include proof of all licenses, certifications and any other information requested by such official.

2. The Hospital's Vice President for Nursing must certify that the applicant has been credentialed as a Special Health Nursing Professional at the Hospital. This certification shall be submitted by the Faculty NP with his/her application.

3. Each Faculty NP who wishes to apply for admitting privileges must be recommended for the granting of admitting privileges by the Dean of the Columbia University School of Nursing who must certify that the applicant is a member of the School of Nursing faculty. The recommendation and certifications shall be submitted by the Faculty NP with his/her application.

4. Each Faculty NP applying for admitting privileges shall obtain from the Director of each Service of the Hospital to which each is seeking admitting privileges all written agreements and protocols governing the Faculty NP's practice and shall submit such documents with his/her application.

• • • • •

The Presbyterian Hospital
in the City of New York
Columbia - Presbyterian Medical Center
New York, NY 10032 - 3784

DATE ISSUED	NUMBER
ISSUED MAY 4, 1994	12.9402

APPROVED	PAGE
MEDICAL BOARD 4/20/94	3 OF 3

MEDICAL BOARD
POLICY AND PROCEDURE MANUAL

5. The Senior Vice President for Medical Affairs shall submit
the application and all relevant materials to the Medical
Board for its review and consideration. Approval by the
Medical Board shall complete the application process.

6. A Faculty NP who is granted admitting privileges shall
function at all times in accordance with his or her practice
agreements, written protocols, delineation of privileges and
the Policies and Procedures of the Medical Board.

Lewis P. Rowland, M.D.
President, Medical Board

William T. Speck, M.D.
President

● ● ● ● ●

But this was only the beginning. Many questions arose, most significantly, "What does an NP need to know to admit and manage a hospitalized patient?" and, "How can they attain these additional skills?" Concurrent with this critical skill development period, we needed to work closely with hospital nursing so that the new NP authority could be implemented—we needed them to care for our patients. And we had another overwhelming piece of the project to establish at the same time: developing and funding the sophisticated evaluation we knew was fundamentally important. We didn't want to lose this opportunity to make a national impact. I don't think it occurred to us that the findings of the study would be anything but positive.

We began 1994 with nearly everyone on the faculty involved in an aspect of the new and innovative faculty practice project. We initially focused on working with our medical colleagues to identify and teach additional skills the NPs might require for the new full-scope practice. It was determined that

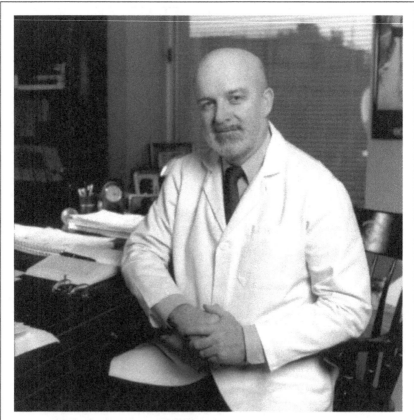

William Speck, MD, president of Presbyterian Hospital (1993)
One of our heroes.

● ● ● ● ●

the NPs would go through a 3-month training period in the Department of Medicine and would be individually credentialed for new procedures through the medical board. The chairman of medicine, Mike Weisfeldt, oversaw the process, which was intensive and comprehensive. The NPs would engage in medical residency education for specific learning in reading imaging studies, interpreting complex and advanced lab results, and performing differential diagnostic work with complex patients.

The hospital was responsible for obtaining funding from New York State to finance the new practice, and we, in the school, held financial responsibilities for the education of the NPs, for startup funds for costs related to faculty, and for the evaluation. The New York State Department of Health funding expected by the hospital for NP salaries did not initially come through. There was some disagreement about whether the hospital or school would supply those missing funds; Bill Speck came to the rescue and committed hospital funds. Choosing space was another issue; the hospital offered space we believed was inadequate (stacked trailers was a June 1994 option) and different from space offered the physicians in our planned comparative study. There were several delays and new options until, in December, I stated in a letter "I will not move the practitioners" to a site unless it was comparable in space. We finally settled on offices near the community hospital site of Presbyterian some 12 blocks north of the medical center. The MD comparison practice was to be in a similar location.

ESTABLISHING THE INPATIENT ADMITTING PROGRAM

Three faculty members who had successful practices at Presbyterian Hospital took the lead in working with nursing at Presbyterian to set the stage for our inpatient admitting program: Penny Buschman (psych), Jennifer Dohrn (midwife), and Patty Ruiz (pediatrics), all of whom were well known and respected by Presbyterian nurses. Their outreach was welcomed by the nursing staff, whom we knew would be the critical link in successful NP management of inpatients. It was determined that the best way to start would be to identify dedicated beds (a particular unit in the hospital) where faculty NPs would admit their adult patients; pediatric patients would be admitted to Babies Hospital and midwifery patients to the Presbyterian satellite community hospital, the Allen Pavilion. This allowed us to focus our attention on a manageable number of staff and administrative nurses. Our faculty liaisons did a great job in securing strong partnerships on adult, pediatric, and obstetrics units. As the scope of inpatient authority was determined and taught in the medical school to our NPs, the nurses on those designated units were kept informed and helped our "resident" NPs learn the ropes. The NPs, many of whom had never worked at Presbyterian, spent time side by side with their Presbyterian nurse colleagues to understand the interchange of staff nurse/attending clinician responsibilities. This was, in fact, our first accomplishment in developing the new practice.

We then began the process of negotiating the NP's withdrawal from their current practices. The new roles would entail being on-call evenings, nights, and weekends, but the heightened faculty interest in joining the new team made these issues easier to resolve. We followed our tried-and-true, 8-year-old faculty practice contracts, with adjustments in outpatient hours to accommodate time expected to be spent in on-call or hospital activities. The new practice was first scheduled to open in the fall of 1994; the faculty NPs used the summer months before that date to learn the new clinical skills and knowledge they would need for inpatient comanagement. We didn't know whether an NP's scope of practice would be sufficient for inpatient management. Perhaps some patients were hospitalized to have a better-monitored care environment, one that might be mandated by the urgency or instability of a chronic illness. For example, a new or unstable diabetic might need hospital monitoring to reach equilibrium, or someone in early heart failure might need diuresing in a hospital environment. But even then, we asked ourselves, wouldn't we want an endocrinologist or cardiologist co-managing a patient in such an urgent state? We couldn't envision a necessary hospitalization that wouldn't entail our request for a specialist consult. And we knew many projected hospitalizations might simply require a referral to a specialist—a surgeon, a neurologist, a cardiologist, or others. Nonetheless, we believed there was value (beyond a comparability research study) to NP hospital admitting privileges.

When a patient is hospitalized, the focus of care is usually on a narrow medical diagnosis. If the admission is unplanned, the patient or his family may not remember or have an opportunity to relate important information, such as medications the patient is taking, or important social aspects of the patient's life. He may be, for example, the sole caregiver of a severely compromised spouse or parent, may abuse alcohol or drugs, or may have had a long-ago medical episode now forgotten, but very relevant to his current illness. A patient's primary care clinician may remember all of these things and may be the educated eyes and ears to help coordinate, order tests, and monitor a hospitalization that could otherwise go awry. There is another value to admitting privileges for primary care clinicians, particularly nurses caring for patients with chronic illnesses. If hospitalization becomes necessary because of a chronic illness crisis or instability, being intimately involved with the admission and care gives the clinician far more influence postdischarge in helping patients more effectively follow preventive care regimens, and understand in a real-time way how the patient responded to treatment. Being otherwise captive to an office encounter robs the clinician of crucial information needed to properly manage a chronic illness or unstable disease.

Another benefit of admitting privileges is knowing when to discharge a patient. Elderly individuals or patients with fragile health may do far better if they can be discharged from a hospital as soon as possible if they have appropriate care at home. The financial imperatives for hospitals already favor early discharge, but who knows better where recovery can best occur than the clinician who recalls how the patient thrived before the current hospitalization? A primary care clinician with access and authority for hospitalizing patients is often a very cost-effective asset for hospitals and for specialists who may have no prior knowledge for a patient's resources, usual health, or ability to care for himself.

In the summer of 1994, the NPs joined medical residents as they learned about radiology, cardiology, orthopedics, sophisticated differential diagnostic skills, and emergency room (ER) evaluations. By shadowing a physician colleague, they learned informally how to admit and co-manage hospitalized patients. The faculty NPs knew from their own professional experience how multitiered inpatient care tends to be, but now they had to figure out whom to call, when, and for what, and how to exert the authority so that necessary responses would be forthcoming. It was daunting for faculty NPs, but as they look back on those days they remember having great confidence and facing the new challenge with excitement. Their training—and the professional relationships with the physicians who would help them co-manage their hospitalized patients—was a magnificent success.[1] In addition to the faculty training and privileges, which demanded so much work, and the careful partnership development with hospital nursing, we also had faculty working on other projects:

- How could we get recognition for their new responsibilities from other hospital departments including lab and radiology staff?
- Could we include student education in this innovation?
- And, importantly, could we obtain funding to support our scientific evaluation of this broad new enterprise?

We spent many hours planning to ensure that the faculty in the new CAP would be equitably compensated for their extended hours (call, hospital rounds, ER, holiday coverage). They kept logs on their time spent in the hospital seeing their patients or responding to patients during their on-call hours. We wanted to quantify how much extra time was spent outside of the office practice. As might be expected, the extra hours were sporadic and not easily forecasted, so the faculty in the practice simply filled in for each other and took the time needed to fulfill their new responsibilities. They functioned as a true team practice. Because we wanted to compare MD/NP productively, we tried to keep practice days separate from teaching days. Some of the practitioners wanted to fit in teaching a 2-hour class on a practice day by not scheduling patients during the 2 hours. In a mature practice that might have worked, but when we were counting the number of patients per NP in each day of practice, it would have been a confounding variable. CAP practitioners were all part time in practice, even though each day devoted to practice was a full day. The remaining percent of their full-time appointment was devoted to teaching or other academically based responsibilities. The MDs in the corresponding practice were all full time. While no formal accommodation in salary was made for inpatient admitting/follow-up, we did increase salary proportionately for holiday coverage and on-call responsibilities.

This new model caused concern among faculty in other practices and among nonclinical faculty who also devoted extraordinary time to their research, including evenings, weekends, and holidays. This was a very sensitive development, and even with a clear focus and communication there emerged a sense within the faculty that CAP was receiving preferential attention. Transparency in our deliberations and decisions helped smooth these concerns, but they did not fully abate and indeed they were correct; the CAP practitioners were front and center, but they also held far more professional burdens and risks than others.

The year before our new practice opened, the New York State attorney general had determined that NPs certified in the state had the "authority independently to prescribe drugs, including controlled substances." The federal Drug Enforcement Administration, relying on this interpretation, has since issued individual registration number to New York State NPs giving them authority to prescribe independently. This authority opened a new scope of practice, although they had been well educated in pharmacology and medication treatment of diseases.

Nurse practitioners have been a highly influential group in arguing for less regulation. They argue that informal practice changes are already in place and that policy should catch up and authorize these advancements. In fact, policy often follows where practice has already arrived, and it rarely dictates new authority ahead of the demand to recognize what has already been established. Certificates in clinical specialties, for example, are established after new competencies have already been learned by a significant number of its members. Certification usually requires evidence of competency and may require prescribed educational achievements for those who follow. Unlike certification, in regulatory advancement that crucial quality step is often omitted—the one that requires evidence of competency before new authority for practice at a new level. The authority to prescribe all drugs came with the stroke of a pen, with no added requirements other than already being approved by the state as an NP. This unsupported regulatory authority would happen again in 1997 when the balanced budget amendment entitled NPs to direct reimbursement for care of Medicare patients *in any site of care*: NPs were not then—or now—educated to provide care in all settings.

Nurses, eager to achieve regulatory approval for practice already widely established, have not advocated a regulatory step that would initially require competency testing for the new level of practice. Our profession has not done so for advancing prescriptive authority or for eliminating MD supervision in many states. They are winning the unilateral arguments to reduce restrictive regulations with little evidence. Why is nursing winning? Not necessarily because policy makers trust nursing's self-serving statements, but because of the public's overwhelming and unmet need for services. We in nursing should not be so willing to accept regulatory advancements without requiring standards of competency and excellence. As we are winning the battles to reduce regulation, we should understand the reason this is happening, and not delude ourselves that we have done enough until we demand competency evidence and standards to accompany all regulatory release. If not, we embrace a profession sadly lacking in responsibility to patients and accountability for our practice.

Certainly the New York State policy authorizing independent drug prescribing helped us as we planned our comparability study a year later. Our practitioners were diligent in their individual efforts to learn about drugs new to their scope of practice. This I know because of discussions in the Faculty Practice Committee. But we made no efforts to advocate for New York State standards of competency in this area for NPs.

EVALUATING CAP: THE NP–MD COMPARABILITY STUDY

In 1994, as we planned the study comparing NPs and MDs, the knowledge required for the NPs' new level of practice was carefully taught in a specially designed summer residency, overseen by the hospital medical board, and chairs in the medical school. Later, when we contemplated how to change regulatory policy to allow other NPs to achieve the independent primary care practice we had developed, we used the evidence from the randomized trial with Medicaid patients (CAP) and the operational success of the broader practice (Columbia Advanced Practice Nurse Associates [CAPNA]) which was based on the same educational preparation. But as history would show, our two-dimensional approach—meant to link competency with policy—would not be easy.

On July 1, a New York State grant finally came through to the hospital to fund the startup costs for the new NP practices and to fit out the space selected for the practice. The school received a grant from the Leslie Samuels and Fan Fox Foundation for an evaluation of the practice. The executive director of the foundation (Mo Katz) asked us to appoint "hostile" advisors to make sure we addressed all possible issues in our plan. We did not project costs or income to the school for two reasons. First the financial risks were unknown. There were no data available on net profit or loss from an independent NP primary care practice. Second, the hospital was funded for the clinic establishment, so the risk was theirs. Our evaluation would tell whether NP practices could be cost effective.

By May it was clear that we could not utilize faculty midwives in our new plan. New York State had passed a law requiring new, higher standards for midwifery education, but non-nurse midwives would be grandfathered in and would include those practicing at Presbyterian without master's degrees. Because of the diversity in hospital midwives' training, many were not even educated as nurses and the hospital had therefore imposed limitations on the overall scope of midwifery practice in the hospital. These limitations were unacceptable to our faculty midwives and would have compromised an evaluation comparing physician and NP practice in obstetrics.

We had been developing and submitting several grants to fund the evaluation of CAP. By the beginning of May, we were awaiting responses from the Department of Health of New York State; the Division of Nursing, Bureau of Health Professions, Health Resources, and Service Administration; the Kellogg Foundation; and the Macy Foundation. Meanwhile, we had recruited an outstanding group of professionals who agreed to serve as advisors on the planning grant.

- Linda Aiken—a leading nurse researcher at the University of Pennsylvania prominent for her workforce evaluations
- Paul Cleary—an eminent Harvard researcher known for his work on costs and outcomes
- Arnold Epstein—a physician known for his outcomes research
- Tom Inui—a Harvard clinician scientist
- Sherry Glied—a Columbia public health researcher involved in cost analysis of clinical practice

THE FIRST ELECTRONIC HEALTH RECORD AT COLUMBIA

We also received a grant from Hewlett-Packard to establish an online patient care record. We were ahead of the medical center in considering an electronic record, and therefore communications between physicians/lab or x-ray technicians and our NPs were not initially possible using an electronic record. But what this *did* do was allow our NPs to communicate easily with each other regarding care and tests and plans for patients. This was especially important for a practice such as ours, where all the practitioners were part time, requiring careful communication to provide seamless care.

LIABILITY AND MALPRACTICE COVERAGE

Although Speck had initially written me that the hospital would provide full malpractice insurance for CAP providers, his staff was not always up to date with his promises. He always bootstrapped them into his promised support, but they often viewed the many innovative aspects of this project with surprise and wariness. In June, we were still discussing malpractice insurance with the hospital and with Columbia University's legal counsel.

The outcome of these discussions was that the employer—which was the hospital for CAP and for its MD practices—would pay malpractice insurance premiums. The individual practitioners would each continue to hold their own policy, but it would be secondary to the hospital's coverage. Our concern in the school of nursing was with the entrepreneurial scope of the new practices and with the guarantee I wanted to give faculty that they would not be personally liable for potentially problematic outcomes of newly approved activities. And I wanted to be sure the school's growing—and precious— endowment would not be at risk from a legal suit against our faculty. We received assurances that faculty with their own policy plus the hospital policy would be provided with all the coverage needed and that any successful liability suit against our practice would "hit the university endowment, not the school endowment." In a letter from Columbia University's legal counsel dated June 24, 1994, we were advised to go forward with our plan, and that the university stood by us.

IMPLEMENTING THE LARGER PLAN

On June 1, we were working with a plan to complete the following:

1. Facility (construction, architects, patient flow, storage, patient waiting area, etc.)
2. Integrations (medical records, operational procedure)
3. Personnel—the biggest issue, which most of all had to address the assurance of continuity and prevention of gaps in care since CAP providers would be part-time practitioners—and part-time teaching faculty. We had never before run our own 24/7 practice, with the accountability, staff, access, and communications this entailed.
4. Evaluation and funding: We wanted to identify what full scope, crosssite practice looked like, what it accomplished, and how this compared to conventional MD care.

Working closely together, the CAP pioneers—eight in all—worked with their medical colleagues to develop an educational program.

Without the superb and insightful direction of Mike Weisfeldt, chairman of medicine, identifying content training would have been a minefield for us. Weisfeldt was the strongest advocate during these heady days of the new and fragile project, and would continue to be through the establishment of CAP, and even the more contentious CAPNA practice that would follow. He won the day for us, with the Medical Board admitting privileges, making our joint innovation appear safe, reasonable, and the very thing prestigious medical centers are uniquely qualified to do. He even hired a lawyer specifically to work on this issue. When the New York State Medical Association raised their collective eyebrows, he quashed their concerns with sublime assurance that this was appropriate and legal and that many Medicaid patients could not otherwise receive access to care.

Many of our MD colleagues, who believed as we did that NPs have a distinctive and useful approach to primary care, pushed me mercilessly to stop comparing NPs with MDs and instead just show the extent of NP distinctive practice. While agreeing with their observation—NP primary care is distinctive—the overriding reason to show MD comparability was both political and financial. Without comparable outcomes, there would be no comparable reimbursement or comparable public acceptance. Only after securing comparability would the distinctive nature of NP practice have added value; prevention of illness or disease consequences, a higher level of competent self-care for patients, broad and knowledgeable use of community resources—especially for families of patients—all these quality and cost-reducing approaches and strategies make NP practice the *preferred* practice *as well as* a practice comparable to conventional medicine. For me it was not a difference of opinion on these important distinctions, but a

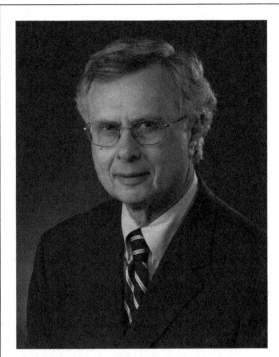

*Mike Weisfeldt, MD, chairman of medicine,
Columbia's College of Physicians and
Surgeons. Another of our heroes.*

• • • • •

difference of priority as to when to address them. Politically I believed that comparability had to come first.

Interestingly, this same conflict (distinctiveness or sameness) was still an issue 15 years later as we try—still—to obtain pay and authority equity for Doctors of Nursing Practice (DNP). Many physician friends are still advocating that we focus on the distinct excellence of DNP rather than MD comparability. Both of course are necessary, and the primary political effect of attempting to convince the public of both has occupied my interest and efforts these many years.

ESTABLISHING THE SCOPE OF THE 3-YEAR RESEARCH STUDY

Our initial draft for a research study opined that a case control study would emerge, and hypothesized that nurses in the study, as compared with physicians, would:

- Spend more time with patients
- Provide more preventive care and counseling
- Develop more elaborate plans for health promotion and symptoms management
- Order fewer tests, procedures, medications
- Consult more often with other practitioners
- Have a lower rate of hospital admissions

Clearly we were being influenced by those who wanted us—in this unique opportunity—to show that nurses had a *distinctive* practice. But this was fraught with danger. If we spent more time and consulted more often, we would not be a preferred financial model. And while health promotion, disease prevention, and more time with patients might be a good thing, these activities were not reimbursable and would not be influential in achieving par reimbursement or equal authority to provide care. The study design remained unfinished.

At the end of the summer all of our funding requests were either being considered or had been awarded; there was great excitement about evaluating CAP as a national model. The plan we finally developed was a randomized controlled trial—the first ever done comparing NPs with physicians. This trial became possible for two reasons. First, we had the dedicated help of Bob Kane in doing it right, and we had an MD practice for comparison. Kane is a physician, university administrator, and a distinguished health services researcher at the University of Minnesota, who gave generously of his time, knowledge, and guidance. He became a regular member of our working group, tutoring us, cajoling us, challenging us to get it right. Second, the hospital was opening, for the first time, a family practice residency. It was set to welcome the first residents and codirectors, on July 1, 1994, just weeks before CAP would open.

This provided a fresh MD practice—recruiting new patients just as CAP would do—and at the same time. This could provide us with an unparalleled opportunity to compare very similar practice environments, with the only difference being professional preparation: MD or NP. This opportunity disappeared when the new family practice physicians failed to get admitting privileges. It was ironic that our nurses could admit, but not family practice physicians. We found the appropriate comparison group of MDs in the hospital's Ambulatory Care Network Corporation (ACNC)—a broad constellation of hospital clinics (CAP was one) serving the community need for care.

Bob Kane guided us through the planning, conduct, and analysis of this 3-year effort. His work with us was undeniably the strongest and most critical aspect of a successful and high-quality study. During the summer of intense residency training so that CAP nurses could begin practice September 1, our evaluation team planned and structured the research design and the activities in support of the study. Nearly every faculty member in the school had a role in this project paving the way with nurse colleagues at the hospital, developing practice and operational protocols, recruiting patients, participating in the residency, and working on our several funded projects. It was a very exciting and cohesive period of achievement in the school. A work plan for all of these activities, from July through September, lists 34 separate activities for which someone was responsible. I don't think anyone had a "summer vacation." In June, the Macy Foundation grant, "A Collaborative Approach to Family Practice," was funded for $500,000; the Health and Human Services division of nursing approved a 5-year grant written by Terry Doddato "to improve models of primary care" for over $1 million, real money in those days.

All of the letters from Bill Speck beginning January 1994 until CAP opened allude to the "exciting and unique" project we were conducting. It was a time of shared trust and cooperation with the hospital that had been long hoped for. This was possible because—finally—the hospital had a need that could make use of our major resource, advanced practice nurses, and because we had the superb, brave, and visionary support of Bill Speck.

On July 18, I wrote a long letter to faculty, alumni, and our growing band of advocates. While praising the research and policy eminence in the school, which were increasingly achieving national attention, I wrote that "practice is the heart of our investigations and the soul of what we hope to improve." In this same letter I noted the promotion of Sarah Cook to senior associate dean, with responsibilities of "authority for the day-to-day functioning of the school." In this letter to colleagues in July, the focus was on embedding our practice initiatives in the center of our research program and solidifying our innovative degree programs, the ETP for college graduates entering nursing, and the Doctor of Nursing Science (DNSc) program in health services research. I believed the overwhelming effort of our new full-scope primary care practice would only have a lasting impact if we conducted a rigorous concurrent evaluation. My letter states, in part, "I believe our faculty resources could take us to the very top of nursing leadership in health services research. We should hold our own in this. We cannot meet that preferred outcome without distinguished practice. Our challenge is to find the balance that will make us more productive."

Columbia's new focus on health services research—conventionally a School of Public Health domain—gained stature by its presence in a clinical practice school. We were finding our balance.

In devising the startup and incremental numbers of practitioners in the new practice, a spreadsheet from July 1994 shows that we started with 3.4 full-time equivalents (eight faculty members), increasing to 4.4 after 9 months. We appointed one NP (Patty Ruiz) to be the lead practitioner, responsible for seamless coordination. In time, we realized that having only part-time practitioners made optimum coordination difficult. Regardless of the faculty members' devoted communications, there were simply too many pending lab results, or expected follow-up appointments (sometimes with a different practitioner because of staffing patterns) and specialist referral responses to be accommodated by a band of part-time faculty. There were no quality or clinical gaps identified because of this model in our first independent practice, and therefore we continued to use that model in the practice we opened in midtown Manhattan 3 years later. Only over time did we realize that the timely and complete care we aspired to was far more likely to happen if we had at least one full-time practitioner overseeing the practice.

The initial salaries for the new practice were in the $60,000 range for 12 months. This was somewhat lower than researcher salaries. I added a bonus of $3,000 for CAP practitioners during the first year because of the extra study and meetings necessary to get the practice established. One of the trickiest planning tasks was to schedule academics for part of their time on an academic schedule and part of their time taking calls on weekends and holidays, and continuing to practice when their nonpractice colleagues were enjoying academic breaks in their routines. We were eroding the traditional "clinical faculty" role and substituting one that was far more attuned to clinical practice priorities. Most faculty were accustomed to academic schedules and scholarly requirements (often conducted during breaks in their teaching schedule) but had once been practitioners engaged in the very different rhythm of patient care. Now they had to do both, often within awkward timing constraints. Thankfully they addressed this challenge with cooperation and optimism.

We included pediatric nurse practitioners (and pediatric patients) within CAP, and it was a vibrant part of the practice. The pediatric data, however, were not included in the evaluation. The reason for this was because the MD comparison practice did not have any pediatric patients.

As 1994 came to a close, CAP opened with a flourish. The patients were mostly young Dominican families who were thrilled and grateful to have responsive and capable clinicians caring for them. But this was not a conventional young population; there was a much higher degree of previously undiagnosed and untreated illness. Childhood asthma was rampant, and had largely been "treated" by repeat ER visits. Now these patients with asthma saw our NP faculty—either in the office, or after they arrived in the ER, or occasionally the PNP made a home visit to identify environmental triggers. It was a profound change in how they received their care and how well they learned to prevent many of these episodes. Although not part of the formal trial, our data show that pediatric patients treated at CAP were far less likely to be hospitalized for asthma attacks than other pediatric asthma patients treated in the ER. Diabetes and hypertension—diseases with few symptoms to send individuals for care—were prevalent in significant numbers in the new CAP adult patients. Part of the satisfaction our clinicians immediately found was the difference they could make in these families' health status.

As the new year dawned, CAP visits grew daily with several appointments from ER randomization. We were on our way.

NOTE

1. The best acknowledgment of this occurred 2 years later. The NPs had by then admitted patients regularly to the adult and pediatric services, and our research was capturing the numbers but not the qualitative aspects of the hospital admitting experiences. The Medical Board had approved these privileges for only 2 years—the extent of the research planned. Before that end date arrived, the Medical Board approved NP admitting privileges as a permanent part of its bylaws. Surprised, I asked if they needed any additional data, as I had submitted none. The answer was, "Not necessary. We've been watching."

7

•••••

Research and Centennial Celebrations

•••••

WHILE THE DEVELOPMENT OF THE Center for Advanced Practice (CAP) and designing and running the randomized trial were consuming activities in the 5 years between 1990 and 1995, two equally important activities were occurring: the rapid and breathtaking growth of our research endeavor and the school's Centennial in 1992.

Under the bold leadership of Herb Pardes, the Health Sciences Division was in the process of unwinding its arcane financial structure in relation to the central university. While blunt and messy, the emerging transparency and fairness were heartening to all of us on a campus not only 50 blocks from the Morningside campus, but with a profoundly different constellation of academic rhythm and use of resources.

The School of Nursing was particularly vulnerable during this transformation. Having been financially and academically opaque within the medical school structure for 50 years, approximating its true costs required double estimates—carving out its specific utilization of resources first from the medical school and then from the university. Complicating this new measurement was the context of nursing's new quarters—a mixed-use building with dorm space (for non-nursing students) taking up the majority of the building, but with the school providing refurbishment and maintenance of the common entrance, lobby, and hallways. The hardest argument was determining the school's legitimate assessment of common costs, which was a university budget committee issue, a committee on which I served during those years.

THE DNSc SUPPORTS NURSING RESEARCH

During the 1990–1991 academic year, several landmark accomplishments occurred. The Health Sciences Division and the provost approved the plan for a Doctor of Nursing Science (DNSc) program. This was a major step toward establishing our school as a research entity. This same year, the seed of what would become a pace-setting mission to endow professorships was planted.

59

In December 1990, the university trustees approved the first endowed chair in the School of Nursing, the Centennial chair in Health Policy. This was the first chair in health policy in any nursing school. Under the vibrant leadership of Doris Hansmann, alumna from 1943 who chaired the school's Centennial Campaign, $500,000 was raised for the $1 million Anna Maxwell Chair in Research, and a challenge grant of $250,000 was received from Sandoz Research Institute toward the $1 million endowed chair in pharmaceutical research. This was possible because Bob Levy, MD, the new CEO of Sandez, had been vice president for Health Sciences at Columbia when I first joined the nursing faculty (and had recommended me for the health policy fellowship at Robert Wood Johnson).

OTHER ACADEMIC SUCCESSES

The Entry to Practice (ETP) program was thriving. Our ability to attract men (20% of the class) and minorities (24%) was excellent. Because most students had been in the workforce, parental financial contributions were nearly nonexistent, and the students' own savings were not nearly enough for the 60-credit 1-year program. The tuition, room, and other essentials came to nearly $90,000 for the year. Our financial aid bill rose to 30% of all revenues, making the ETP program a much smaller contributor to revenues. These students continued seamlessly into the MS phase of their education, thereby continuing their need for financial aid. The hospital subsidies, however, and faculty practice, a major shift to full-time enrollments and extraordinary fundraising allowed the school to thrive financially.

By 1991 only five faculty from 1986 remained, and three of those five were in leadership positions in the school. All other faculty were new recruits. Faculty salaries had increased three times over their 1986 salaries. New research and practice requirements demanded a breadth of skills that former faculty had not developed. The new faculty, dedicated to their research or practice, were remaking the school.

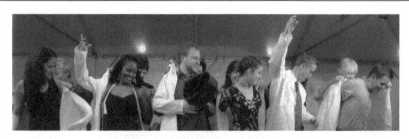

White Coat Ceremony for ETP graduates as they complete their first professional degree in nursing (1995).

• • • • •

However, only 3% of faculty were underrepresented minorities: a dismal proportion then and now. The new generation of nursing faculty—graduates of ETP and then doctoral programs like ours—will certainly be better represented across all cultures and races. During 1991 we strengthened our joint degree with the School of Public Health and developed a new joint degree—MS/MBA—with the Columbia Business School.

THE 1992 CENTENNIAL CELEBRATION

The Centennial event of 1992 gave us an unusually good opportunity to build bridges with the Alumni Association, with whom we hoped to celebrate the school's rich history and with the alumni who made it great. The major reason to heal the hegemony with the old alumni association was not about their funds. The challenge was to establish a united group of alumni for the future. We tried repeatedly to develop a plan whereby the association could continue to keep all their current funds in a private account (they currently use Brown Brothers Harriman) for which they would have sole authority. As part of the plan, the old association would merge with the new one and work in concert on behalf of the school and its students as well as our alumni. They were offered board seats and administrative positions in the blended organization in the same numbers as the new organization leadership. The old association would cease to exist except to manage their original fund. We were fighting for the hearts and minds of our alumni, but the old association's continued inflammatory—and untrue—accusations that we just wanted their money prevented unification and caused alumni to withdraw completely. I also believe that giving $25 a year to their alumni association was far less challenging to older alumni than the prospect that I would expect significant monetary and political support in the new organization. They simply weren't prepared for or interested in that transition. The old alumni association never responded to our proposal, even after we met to discuss it in person with them. The dissonance continued.

THE COLUMBIA MODEL: THE FOUR Ps

We began to think of our initiatives as the Columbia model: the four "Ps":

1. Faculty **Practice**
2. **Precepting** by hospital nurses
3. **Partnerships,** which gave hospitals a guaranteed graduate to hire in return for tuition support
4. New **Pathways** in one nursing program for college graduates

The nursing shortage and resulting bump up in salaries made nursing a more attractive career and gave hospitals the incentive to invest in educating these future professionals. In 1991, this model came into full operation. With the last graduation from the traditional baccalaureate program, we became an all-graduate school, with students whose backgrounds mirrored those in medicine, public health, and dentistry. This accomplishment gave us peer status—our students looked like other health sciences school students, and our faculty looked like other health sciences school faculty. We were coming of age.

A university retreat for Columbia deans late in 1991 provided a rare opportunity to discuss how our schools were addressing the serious financial situation in the university. While nursing's finances were strong and our endowment had reached $16.5 million (adding $6 million in 1991), many schools were dipping into their endowments to meet their expenditures, and the schools that were most successful in building a strong financial base were investing heavily in fundraising. The law school that year had 22 people in its development office, and the business school had nine—including four professors who worked full time raising money. The nursing school stood out as a school with stunning growth of revenues and a strong financial footing, and we saw the Centennial as a rare opportunity to build an even stronger fundraising base.

We continued to deliberate on how to best plan for a new building for nursing. Our growing endowment and unspent revenues were the major source of funding this plan. Other schools in the university had built new buildings or added to their existing one through two avenues: gifts or borrowing money from the university, with expected future revenues pledged to pay off the debt. Usually it took a combination of gifts and debt to pay for the planned building. We thought we could do this. We were then—and continued to be—very careful and conservative with our expenditures. We consistently ended each year with unrestricted unspent revenues, often totaling as much as 30% to 50% of our expenditures. In other words, our expenditures for the year might total $4 million, but we might have $2 million in revenues remaining when all the bills were paid. We were certain we could continue this successful pattern, building a reputation as a worthy and reliable debtor when it came time for us to pay for a building. We also were gaining success in our fundraising; this, plus our saved annual revenues, was fast becoming a large nest egg for building our new home.

Financial problems continued to be a major concern for the university in 1991. In December, the *New York Times* ran a front page article, "As a Deficit Looms, 26 Threaten to Quit Key Columbia Posts." All 26 department heads in the arts and sciences threatened to resign if further budget cuts were imposed. The new provost, Jonathan Cole, was quoted as responding, "We've got to be leaner and meaner," including the costs of benefits. On the health sciences campus, our renegotiated fair share of costs—through the common cost assessment—was a significant part of Pardes's remarkable negotiations for the four schools. This could not have happened at a better time to secure the legitimate growth of the Health Sciences Center.

NURSING'S IMPROVED FINANCIAL STATUS

In a 5-year (1985–1990) comparison submitted to Pardes, nursing's annual financial status had changed dramatically:

- Endowment had grown from under $2 million to $10.5 million
- Research had grown from $0 to $489,259 a year
- Annual gifts had grown from $115,000 to $500,000 a year
- Hospital Partnership revenues totaled $549,840 (all placed in the new building fund)
- Faculty Practice revenues were $257,000 a year
- Financial aid grew from $700,000 to $1,282,000 a year

Our contribution to the university for common costs was $948,000, which was over 28% of our revenues and the highest revenue percentage of any of Columbia's 16 schools. This glaring inequity was the only one not resolved by Pardes's restructuring of the health sciences finances. My budget submission to the university trustees on March 6, 1991, stated, "our major expense, and necessary component of our future planning is the critical need for a new building." This was a theme in each of the first 5 years, and thereafter, as our intellectual, professional, and physical presence was limited by an inadequate, decrepit, multiuse building.

THE CENTENNIAL CELEBRATION TAKES SHAPE

The year of our Centennial in 1992 was star-studded and extremely successful, as we engaged old friends in our new endeavors and added substantially to our growing cadre of supporters.

It was a particularly promising year for our outreach to the Alumni Association. While the association remained cautiously independent and continually wary of our plans to engage them, they didn't want to miss being part of the big celebration. The new president of the association, Keville Frederickson, was sincerely interested in building stronger bonds with the school. She was doctorally prepared, unlike former presidents, had a broader and educated view on the school's future, and was a professor at Teacher's College, our Columbia affiliate. She maneuvered her group into supporting part of two endowed chairs, joined in an alumni cruise at sunset on the Hudson, and accepted one of our Centennial awards at the gala. Once the centennial was over, however, the association returned to its sole isolated function and communications essentially ended, except for their check once a year from interest in a few funds in their endowment that were specifically designated for student scholarship at Columbia. This annual check was about $70,000, representing 1% of their endowment, which was then close to $7 million.

+ LDM

MISSIONARIES OF CHARITY
54A A.J.C. BOSE ROAD
CALCUTTA — 700016

Oct 29, ' 91

Dr Mary Mundinger , Dean
School of Nursing
Columbia University
New York, United States.

Dear Dr Mary Mundinger,

This brings you, the staff and the students
of Clumbia Nursing School, my prayer for
God's blessing on your school during this
year of its centennial celebrations. Let
us thank God for all the care that has
been given over the past 100 years through
those trained in your Nursing school.
That is God's gift to you.

I am most grateful to you for your kind
decision to give me the Award. I am sorry
I would not be able to come to receive
the award personally as at that time we
will be having the Professions of our
Sisters here. But I shall be with you all
in prayer that you teach your student-
nurses not only to give their hands to
serve the sick, but also their hearts to
love the suffering, that you make this
Centenary year a year of greater love for
one another and of greater compassion.

God bless you
Me Teresa mc

*Mother Teresa's response to receiving a Columbia Centennial Award
for Excellence (1992).*

● ● ● ● ●

Nonetheless, the Centennial year was an unusual opportunity to bring all of our alumni close to the school, and to begin the significant fundraising necessary to secure our plans for the future. I had seen clearly that the insufficient financial grounding—the permanent kind—not just an annual year in the black, was the best bulwark against onslaughts that were all too common against nursing schools. Our rupture with the hospital was a necessary adolescent independent move, but we essentially left our material legacy in the hands of our former parent. There was only a bitter inheritance of affront and anger. Moving from the hospital to departmental status in the medical school took us appropriately into the environment of higher education, but the hierarchical and paternalistic attitude toward medicine and nursing hardly fostered our independence. Interestingly, it was the university and the public's conventional view of medical dominance over nursing that was far more apparent than that of our own medical faculty. Nonetheless, as a department—not a school—nursing could not fully develop an independent presence. This constraining structure was in place from 1937 until I became dean in 1986—nearly 50 years longer even than our initial 45 years as a hospital school. Wrenching full school status from the university required support from Herb Pardes—one of his many gifts to the school—and the concerted efforts of the dean of Public Health, Allan Rosenfield, who was pushing for the same independence for his school. As this played out, in mind-numbing proposals, our centennial provided the timing and rationale to begin a major fundraising effort. Nursing schools with money were far more secure than schools without—even if they had a stellar faculty and hundreds of students. And not just money, but endowment money, is what I believed would anchor our future. The school of nursing at Cornell had been closed by the university because of a deficit of about $500,000 in Cornell's New York Hospital budget. Cornell nursing was part of the hospital then, and the hospital's accounting of the school's revenues and expenses showed the school running a deficit of $500,000. By closing the school, the hospital deficit disappeared. It was an easy decision (based on personal communication with New York Hospital trustee, Byron Saunders). If the school had been independent, with its own budget, it may have made a different accounting, or might have seen the deficit looming and begin to erase it. If it had its own budget and endowment, the outcome might have been different. I was determined to plant the seeds of survival for Columbia nursing by continuing to build our endowment.

CENTENNIAL FUNDRAISING

Doris Hansmann, our campaign chair, was an extraordinarily charismatic and spunky woman. She had not been particularly active as an alum (there was no structure to do so on behalf of the school), but she was willing to take on the daunting challenge of raising $3 million. Considering that

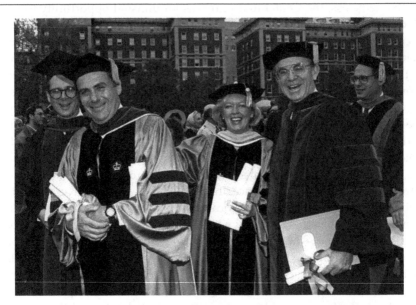

Herb Pardes, MD, dean of Medicine and vice president for Health Sciences (1990) rounding out our triumvrate of heroes. Pictured here with, to his right, Dean Mundinger and Allan Rosenfield, dean of the School of Public Health. Pardes established Public Health and Nursing as independent schools during his tenure.

• • • • •

the Columbia Business School endowment was currently $22 million, our $3 million fundraising goal was breathtaking. Doris and I formed a firm bond and a deep friendship in our work together on Centennial fundraising. One day in a blizzard we arrived on time for an appointment with the CEO of United Parcel Service (UPS). He was surprised we had made it, and Doris laughed and poking her finger in his chest said, "We are always on time— just like UPS." And yes, he gave us money. Even Doris's license plate gave warning about her attitude: ZIPPY. Doris's husband, Ralph, a highly successful business entrepreneur, quietly developed access for us everywhere in New York City. He was our silent influential partner, opening doors and lasting recognition for Columbia School of Nursing. We called him Prince Ralph, our benefactor.

The first major event of our celebratory year was a Health Care Auction. It was held in the heady atmosphere of Christie's. The steering committee included Arthur Ashe, who attended and donated a pair of his tennis shoes which he wore when he won at Wimbledon. The winning bid was only $200, and then, amazingly, the winner did not claim the shoes, which disappeared in the move back from Christie's to Columbia when the auction was over. Someone, somehow, has some iconic and legacy-filled sneakers. The benefit committee was comprised solely of alumni, including Marilyn Hamel, who made a gorgeous quilted panorama of the school's history centered with the figure of Anna Maxwell, which today hangs in the school's alumni offices. Several prominent physicians from current and past Columbia leadership attended and contributed, including Burt Lee, Ed Bowe, David Habif, Louis Bigliani, Lewis Rowland, Don Tapley, Mike Katz, and Frank Stinchfield, who also donated the gift bags. The oldest alumni donor was Marion Cleveland, from the class of 1927. Sixty-seven donors provided auction items ranging from spa days to ski lessons, a weekend ocean house retreat, and health club memberships. The auction netted $33,305. As the Centennial year kicked off, we had already raised $1,118,226. The mark of Ralph Hansmann was on many of the corporate gifts from AT&T, Citicorp, Colgate-Palmolive, IBM, Manufacturers Hanover, Polaroid, Westinghouse, and Xerox. But it was

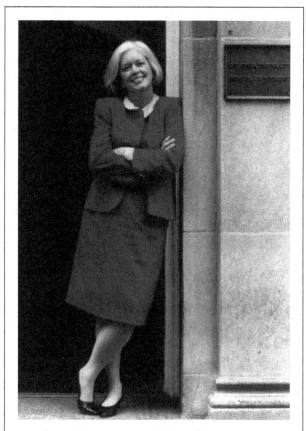

*Dean Mundinger on the day of the school's
Centennial, 1992.*

• • • • •

Doris who personally conveyed the importance of nursing to those corporate executives and brought the gifts home.

The Centennial year was a turning point for the school. Our financial position had stabilized, and we had completed 5 years of growth in resources, endowment, and faculty recruitment. The school gave the first Centennial Awards for Excellence to the association's president Keville Frederickson, Princess Diana, Mother Teresa, and Princess Aga Khan. We held a black-tie event at the St. Regis Hotel in midtown Manhattan. Although many of our alumni bought tables and brought guests, I faced the embarrassing quest of convincing other Columbia deans to buy tables. They demurred, saying "we are all fundraisers" for our own schools and shouldn't be squandering hard-won funds on another dean's school. I was offended to think we deans shouldn't indeed spend for each other and the common good (I had given funds to the hospital annual events for this reason), but I found the only way to get them to our celebratory event was to give them free tickets. At least they came. It may be that the really difficult financial situations in their own schools prevented them from giving to nursing. But this did not change our own values with regard to supporting sister schools in the future (for example, when we commissioned a portrait of our esteemed colleague Allan Rosenfeld as he left the deanship of public health). Maybe nurses just view things differently, but our faculty always provided this kind of support to others in the university. The evening celebrating our Centennial was an exciting one for all of us. We felt that we had truly arrived as members of the larger university, and we reveled in our successes.

These Centennial activities were important for presenting a strong, new, and independent presence in the university, and for catching the interest of thousands of alumni who had never been asked to help and honor their school. Luckily we had this marvelous opportunity to reengage those who had been isolated from the school since their graduation. During the Centennial year, I visited a magnificent woman who had been a colleague of Anna Maxwell, the founder of our school. She was in an assisted living home in Florida and was 98 years old in 1992. She had been a young faculty member with Anna Maxwell, early in the century, and was in France with her when the then Presbyterian Hospital School sent nurses to serve in Europe during the First World War. She said Maxwell was very strict and severe, but a compassionate woman who was devoted to her school and to nursing. Interestingly, she told me that Maxwell spoke with a strong Scottish accent. It was magical to hold the hand of a woman who had served with the woman who established the school 100 years before.

In September, in the welcoming convocation, during our Centennial year, Joseph Califano admonished the students: "It's time to give nurses more to do; get off the sidelines and into the front lines." Columbia nursing was listening and eager to follow his bidding; already brave and innovative, the faculty was on its way to even greater successes and landmark achievements.

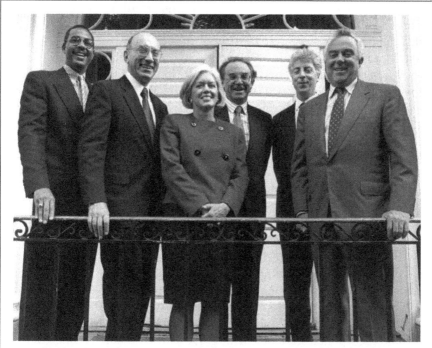

Centennial speaker group. (1991) Left to right: Dr. Reed V. Tuckson, president of Charles R. Drew University of Medicine and Science, Los Angeles; Michael I. Sovern, Columbia University president; Dr. Mary O. Mundinger, dean of the School of Nursing; Dr. Herb Pardes, dean of Medicine and vice president for Health Sciences, Dr. Jonathan R. Cole, university provost; and Joseph A. Califano, Jr.

• • • • •

As 1992 drew to a close, our budget for the following year reflected our continued academic and financial successes. We always projected revenues very conservatively (no new gifts or grants were projected), which meant every new grant or gift was revenue beyond those revenues listed in our proposed budget. We always exceeded our projections. The endowment had grown to $16.7 million, which reflected unspent endowment income for several years, annual transfer of unrestricted revenues remaining after all expenses were paid, and new gifts, particularly to the Maxwell Chair ($870,000), the Alumni Chair ($1 million), and the Pharmaceutical Research Chair ($500,000).

The Doctor of Nursing Science (DNSc) program, newly approved, was gearing up to recruit its first students. We aimed at admitting only full-time students to foster strong relationships with senior faculty and to provide the focused attention required to become a researcher. I had determined that a DNSc degree was preferable to a PhD degree for us at this time. Although the PhD was the ultimate goal—as a more recognizable and accepted academic achievement—I did not think it was advisable as our entry point in doctoral education. At Columbia, all PhD programs are under the aegis of the Graduate School of Arts and Sciences. This unit, on the Morningside campus, was composed of research faculty who knew nothing about academic nursing. A conventional PhD program for nursing would have little chance of incorporating the scholarly attributes of our profession. PhD programs similar to Columbia's PhD program were already available to nurses who wanted to earn a doctorate. Therefore, I believed a doctoral degree that would be developed in a nursing school, determined by nurses, reflected nurses' scholarship, and offered a degree in nursing was the best first step. A later evolution to a PhD would then be more likely to contain the elements of academic nursing than if we chose the PhD as our first doctoral degree program.

Our experience with graduate education—the MS in advanced practice where nearly all students were part time and working in lesser roles—overwhelmingly showed the difficulty in adopting newly independent roles while practicing full time in the old ones. We believed that full-time doctoral education could ameliorate that difficult transition.

The years ahead would show how wrong we were to expect full-time study without significant student funding and without funded research that could incorporate student learning. We learned that part-time graduate study for nurses was a firmly entrenched model, and without significant funding for a student's tuition and research position, our full-time model could not be sustained, nor could it compete with part-time programs elsewhere. Other factors were also at work; nurse salaries were very good and hard to give up for a degree that might not increase one's salary. Another deterrent to full-time study was the fact that most nurses entered graduate education after establishing families and incurring debt. Full-time graduate study was not part of this culture. As we developed teaching assistantships (TAs) and grant supported research assistants (RAs), full-time enrollment for the doctoral students became a reality, but in the early years the applicants were few and poorly attuned to what full-time doctoral study entailed.

While our admission applications reached an all-time high, we were forced to curtail enrollment in the ETP program for college graduates due to a lack of clinical sites. Although we tried to increase our student presence at Presbyterian Hospital, in 1993 they reduced our student clinical placement in positions from 40 to 12, but accepted students from several other schools, including New York University and the University of Pennsylvania where officers of the old Alumni Association were faculty members. Nonetheless, we proposed to the Presbyterian Department of Nursing a partnership to establish a nurse-run clinic. Although this proposition foundered, a different version, emanating from the Presbyterian president's office, had surfaced by the end of the year and would bring us in close alliance with the hospital and their nurses.

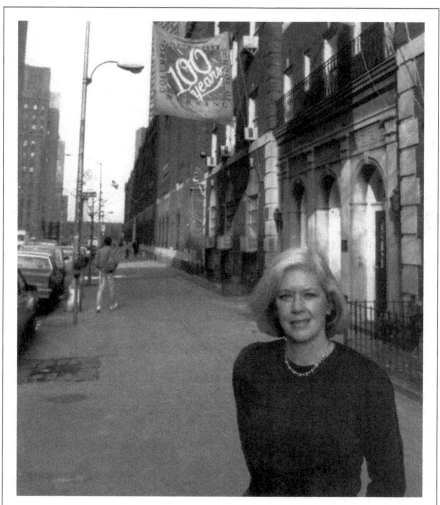

Mary O. Mundinger (1992) at Nursing's home base at the time of the Centennial Celebration.

• • • • •

Much of the conflict between the Presbyterian nursing service and Columbia nursing was conventional service/education conflict territory, especially where university education adopted higher level education programs that no longer focused on preparing hospital bedside nurses. But more was occurring at our medical center, which worsened the normal conflicts. First, the rupture from a hospital-based school to a university entity had never healed. Second, the unipurpose Alumni Association, which never had school support as part of its mission, was totally focused on its own organizational meetings and internal camaraderie, with a minor focus on alumni from the school. Many of the officers of the association were Presbyterian Hospital employees. They cherished the hospital legacy of their education and had been in their positions on the Alumni Association board long before I became dean, and are still there today, over a quarter of a century later. A broadening of the Alumni Association mission to include the school was not possible with the limited vision of its board and their positions at Presbyterian where they fanned the flames of discord.

During 1993, we again made an impassioned plea to the university to help find us a new home in a different and more unifying building. Our budget submission notes: "problems of excessive to insufficient heat; steam leaks, rats, mice, roaches; endless fire alarms (student tenants' toasters and small ovens . . .), inadequate and often broken elevator service, broken windows . . ." and the ever present armory next door which housed 2,000 homeless men.

We continued to build an endowment that could form the basis of paying for a new building. In the interim, the best the university could do was agree to provide an extra guard at the front of the building.

While we struggled with finding the right pattern for doctoral student engagement, we were encountering a growing disparity between doctoral and clinical faculty salaries. Faculty practice salaries were now higher than faculty researchers' salaries and higher than their own academic salary base. We determined that the only fair thing to do (and that we could afford to do) was to raise both research and clinical faculty salaries to be equal to external practice salaries. The resulting salary level for faculty then differed only by rank; all assistant professors earned the same starting salary, and all full professors could reach the same salary levels, based on similar contributions such as scholarly publications, national recognition through awards, or presentations. Grant support was required for researchers, and clinical practice for clinical faculty. We were, bit by bit, building a model of equal standing for faculty prepared in each of these roles.

8

•••••

The Perfect Storm

•••••

OUR POSITION WITHIN A MEDICAL center was instrumental to our successful path to independence. Medical schools need primary care for their patients, but they don't want to deliver it. Our experience was not just a serendipitous opportunity to develop advanced primary care; it also entailed a rigorous evaluation, which is more likely to happen in a medical center context and which was necessary to foster adoption of this new level of practice nationally. A medical center context also gave us an abundance of brilliant helpful specialists who gave us a safe and inviting environment in which to spread our wings and expand our practice. It was critically important that these advancements were made and evaluated on the medical center if they were to lead to lasting policy change and national adoption. With medicine so intimately involved in the evaluation of expanded nursing service, the uniqueness of nursing's contributions in the context of the larger health care environment was clearer. Individual assertive and smart nurse practitioners (NPs) nationally had been wresting new hospital and on-call authority for themselves for years. They had been mentored to learn more and do more, but they didn't represent a movement or carefully crafted programmatic advancement. These pioneering individuals were just that, but their ability to open doors for others, or to formalize how they themselves had succeeded, never happened. But a school of nursing, with a school of medicine, the focused leadership of an esteemed medical center hospital, and a large-scale model carefully tested, could break ground for a lasting change in practice. This was our great benefit.

Having common purpose among professionals from several disciplines is a powerful resource, but it is not sufficient for radical change. There has to be a great gap in need of being filled before the revolution can happen. The primary care shortage was the fuel that ignited the revolution, sustained by the hospital's acute need for a new building to remain competitive.

The third element in support of our major step forward was nursing's ability to serve the Medicaid population. The Medicaid reimbursement for free-standing primary care practices was absurdly low. Even when Medicaid paid somewhat better for institutionally based primary care practices, like ours in the hospital system, it is not competitive. The Medicaid population is not sought after for other reasons as well; these poor people have fewer resources—they are late or absent from appointments because they have inadequate transportation or child care, they are less able to follow medical regimens to keep themselves healthy, they cannot afford optimal or even a minimally good diet, and they have so many social burdens that it is difficult to provide adequate medical care. For all these reasons—but mostly for financial reasons—physicians who might have been alarmed at our advancements were not, because ours was only a practice for "poor people." This has always been so. Although the nurse practitioner role was in its infancy in 1972 (just 7 years after Lee Ford and Henry Silver burst on the scene with this new idea), the federal payer for Medicaid and Medicare authorized NPs for direct reimbursement for care of patients who lived in underserved areas. Where practitioners were abundant—suburban areas, for example—NPs still had to be partnered at some level of dependence with a physician to be reimbursed by Medicare and Medicaid.

Just as a perfect storm sinks boats, so can the elements coincide for a great flood of benefit, as they did for us in 1995: Primary care deficit, low reimbursement, and insightful physicians were willing to support an independent nurse practice. It wasn't easy, but it was a foretold success and exciting for all of us who were involved.

The school's broad successes—finances, student enrollments, new programs, and extremely able researchers who could measure our outcomes—were necessary and influential in the achievements we reached in the mid-1990s, and remain so today. Our bigger challenge in 1995 was to move successfully into a broader and more competitive environment; if our care was good enough for patients who had no alternative for care, would we be good enough for those who did?

WHAT DID ALL THIS MEAN?

Two occurrences from this period stand out—the Centennial, which had a rhythm and time of its own choosing, and the development of cross-site care for our nurse practitioners, which, unlike the Centennial, entailed opportunistic timing.

First, the Centennial. What did that mean for us? It highlighted the fact that we were part of the second-longest established private university School of Nursing—only the University of Michigan was older by 1 year. This achievement pretty much said, "we made it," but we also used it as our first effort at major fundraising. Unfortunately, we had to deal with the chasm between hospital school alumni and university-based alumni, one filled with raw feelings and skepticism. And to add to the burden of such a division, it was the hospital-based alums who were of an age and culture to have the deepest pockets; we needed their financial support, but even more, we needed their collegial support for the future. We did raise a good deal of money, even from the reluctant and wary old Alumni Association, but their isolation gave them status that joining us could never replace; they retreated to their old ideas and nursed their significant endowment. So although we raised a lot of money—and created two endowed chairs—we faced our second century with a split alumni base. The hospital, of course, used this to fan the flames of their entreaty for us to do more to support their mission; hospital nursing that was out of sync with university nursing endeavors, especially at our medical center. I was stymied as to how to resolve this conflict. Even now, I'm not sure that it was possible at that time. Our renewal was too new, too ungrounded, too radical for the hospital nursing leadership to understand, much less support. There was nothing in it for them; they had no vision or plan for utilizing advanced practice nurses or research that were core resources for us. At each turn, where we succeeded in building partnerships with other hospitals, we failed at Presbyterian. The president of Presbyterian Hospital—a physician—Bill Speck—asked us to partner with him in a very new way—running a primary care practice independent from physician oversight, and, at our request, admitting privileges for these pioneers. We succeeded at Presbyterian by moving away from their nursing department.

Unlike the hospital nursing leadership, Speck saw us as a different resource than staff nurses. He saw us as primary care clinicians. He saw no conflict with hospital nursing. And his breezy confidence in us went a long way toward our acceptance by hospital nurses when we admitted our patients. Working with them was our first priority; we knew they were critical to our success. And importantly, the staff nurses did not hold the same class conflict between hospital and university nurses as the nursing leadership did. This is entirely understandable: Hospital nursing leadership had to protect the role of their caregivers, whereas the caregivers themselves were excited about partnering with us, and indeed many were our students as well as practicing nurses.

Admitting privileges was a key ingredient to advancing nurse practitioner outcomes. Most of all it allowed a fuller authority and presence with our patients—they were more likely to see us as complete in our responsibilities, and therefore they gave us more respect and were more likely to follow our recommendations for care and for referrals. We were the real thing if we could do all of what primary care physicians could do. Even though a very small percentage of primary care patients are hospitalized by that clinician, having those responsibilities added gravitas to all that we did and directed. It was a transformation from day jobs in a clinical situation to the potential to provide care in any environment where a patient needed care.

Amazingly, both Bill Speck's and Joe Califano's quotes about nurses moving into the front lines and taking over primary care were spoken 20 years ago! Still we haven't taken action. The cover of *The Academic Nurse* from the summer of 1993 tells it all: who, exactly, is "stupid?"

Clearly, we achieved admitting privileges because it was in the physician's best interests. Yes, they trusted us to do it well, but they invested in that trust because there was a growing gap as to where we could be: the bridge to referrals and the resource for basic primary care.

So much of what we accomplished has been the result of opportunity as well as hard work and vision. But why, 20 years later, are these Columbia achievements just that and nothing more? Why hasn't nursing jumped on board to replicate, advance, and take over? Why such conservatism when the opportunities are ripe and the models in place? We would struggle with this question as the years went by, and the answers are still elusive.

Section III

•••••

CAPNA: 1995–2000

•••••

དཔྱང་ཤུགས།

9
• • • • •

Changing Lanes
• • • • •

PATIENT ENROLLMENT IN THE NURSE practitioner (NP) and MD practices began in late 1995. We were 4 months late, and faculty had withdrawn from their established practices in the preceding summer in order to prepare for the new ones. Bill Speck stood by his word and paid the NP salaries during this extended period. The Medicaid population in northwest Manhattan was deeply underserved: There simply had not been enough clinicians who accepted the meager Medicaid or small private payments for primary care. As a result, with the advent of two new practices opening in the midst of their neighborhood, patient enrollment flourished. Referrals came predominantly from the hospital emergency room (ER) which had been their de facto primary care provider. Patients who arrived at the ER with nonurgent conditions were, randomly, referred to either the MD or NP practice.

Most of our projections of expected patient severity had relied on the comparatively young age of the underserved population, and we expected a low prevalence of severe medical conditions. What we had not recognized was that since the population had been without care for years, their symptom-based ER encounters had not uncovered many serious and chronic illnesses. Whereas typical primary care clinicians admit very few patients to the hospital, our population was different, and our clinicians were tested early and often in hospital admissions, specialist referrals, and complex medical situations. The patients didn't have any medical histories or ongoing care encounters to guide the practitioners. Patients had been largely untreated, with undiscovered problems. In the first week of practice, we had three hospital admissions. Everyone was on alert for the next urgent situation. Because of all the orientation with hospital nursing developed by Penny Buschman and our faculty, the hospital admissions went smoothly. The medical and surgical staff were magnificent in responding and supporting the faculty NPs. The only place our faculty ran into surprise and confusion was the ER, where few of the staff knew about the expanded privileges of nurse practitioners. Nonetheless, the NPs were able to examine their ER patients and admit them when needed.

Our initial efforts to focus our admissions on a designated hospital unit never came to fruition. Patients admitted to the hospital almost always required the additional care of a specialist, so admissions went to those units—orthopedics, cardiology, gastrointestinal, and so on. Primary care and collaboration with other specialists was a great value, but rarely was this solely the reason for hospital admission. Patients needed both. Organ failure, broken bones, or fulminating infection—all of which our NPs' patients experienced—required the wisdom and knowledge of a surgeon or medical specialist, with the primary clinician responsible for a patient's overall health and ongoing care.

We had projected that the populations targeted for our practices would have disproportionate diagnoses of hypertension and diabetes, and the randomized controlled trial (RCT) was designed to do secondary analyses on care and outcomes of these diseases. Our projection was correct, but we did not foresee the volume of subacute illnesses, the toll that asthma took on this population, and the prevalence of other chronic illnesses, including cancer. Clearly, the learning curve for the faculty NPs grew exponentially as enrollments from this patient population grew. This was an entirely different experience from what some conservative (non-Columbia) physicians had sneeringly posited: Anyone—even nurse practitioners—could follow medical protocols in caring for a young, healthy population in primary care.

In 1996, 1 year into the new practice, the RCT was still actively enrolling patients. We didn't know yet what the comparative results would show, but we knew our faculty NPs could manage a full-scope primary care practice. We had a team of three people working full time conducting the trial. Bob Kane continued to lead the effort, making numerous trips to New York: He not only ensured impeccable rigor for the process, but had taught us during the trial how to design it, how to conduct it, how to avoid pitfalls, and how to make sure we were collecting all the available data. There was high national interest in our results. Having established a board of advisors and overseers from a national base, the stage was set. There were no nurses on the advisory board—only physicians and health policy PhDs. We knew that if the findings were positive for nurses, it would be physicians and policy experts who would pose the most skeptical questions: We didn't need nurses touting nursing. If the outcomes were negative for nursing, nurses on an advisory board would be irrelevant.

In February 1996, we were already in the planning stages for an even bigger project. Columbia's Center for Advanced Practice (CAP) had been functioning successfully since it opened. Our confidence in the challenging

CAP had grown. We believed the medical needs of poor people were similar to those in the broader population. Why should we limit our practice to Medicaid?

There had always been a disconnect between acknowledging NP competence when physicians were scarce, but questioning NP competence in the care of individuals where MD resources were plentiful was another story. Was it acceptable, or even ethical, to impose a lower quality care on poor and rural populations? Or was this really a division based on protecting the medical profession's access to high-paying patients? We decided to challenge this disconnect and try to resolve it.

10
•••••

Doing the Right Thing
•••••

THE CENTER FOR ADVANCED PRACTICE (CAP) experiment—even before the comparative statistics were in—was a success. The Presbyterian Hospital Medical Board had made nurse practitioner (NP) admitting privileges a permanent policy, but only for those who were nursing faculty. They trusted the standard we had put in place. The privileges were not linked to our original Medicaid population, but covered all patients we served. There was a lot to consider as we contemplated opening an NP practice for the mainstream of primary care patients. This time—unlike CAP—we would have to fund the startup ourselves: securing a site, paying rent, selecting faculty for the practice, making projections about enrollments (no underserved population of patients waiting in line for us), and most importantly, not knowing if patients with unlimited choice of physician providers would choose us instead. And we knew there would be political issues about nurses competing openly for high-paying patients. Another big question was whether we could get commercial insurance reimbursement.

We figured we could get past all this if—a big if—our physician colleagues were prepared to continue to join ranks with us. Standing with us to serve poor people was an easy and socially valuable thing for physicians to do, even while they were attacked for allowing nurses the expanded privileges developed for CAP. But standing by us—and with us—when we opened a clearly competitive practice for preferred patients had no social justification. Yes, there was still a primary care shortage, but would this innovation gain our physician colleagues' support?

During this period, I was appointed to the Clinton Healthcare Team, a small group of physicians, nurses, and health policy experts invited to critique the plan emerging from First Lady Hillary Clinton's major project to overhaul the nation's health care system. I learned about the challenges of a top-down process when the center of the issues is radical transformation. I knew our own small but radical plan required support from the beginning from every quarter.

I met first with Mike Weisfeldt, chair of Medicine, and discussed our bold plan in early 1996. He thought it had merit, and he was willing to champion it with his department, the Medical Board, and the insurers. Again, he used his influence and his power to argue our case. Actually, Mike doesn't argue. He stated his case as though it was inarguable and simply the right thing to do. His confidence in us and the physicians' confidence in him made this plan possible. Mike knew we were headed for an onslaught by organized medicine—probably the American Medical Association (AMA) and New York State Medical Society—so he again secured outside legal assistance to make sure we didn't fall into any traps. He and I also met with Columbia's legal counsel to assure them this plan was entirely legal and that this department backed us. Mike Shelansky, head of the hospital Medical Board, continued to stand by us. Who knew a pathologist would be among our strongest supporters? I think they were intrigued by the looming fight, believed in this continuing mission, and wanted us to win.

Once the physicians and university were on board (we didn't detail to the university how public the controversy would probably be), we had to convince the payers.

CAPNA

As we tinkered with a name for this new practice, CAP already had an identity—a solid, gold one, and we didn't' think we should confuse things by using that name. The next idea was "The Center for Wellness and Prevention" but it was pallid and empty; it said nothing about giving sophisticated comprehensive care. Then we considered "The Columbia Center for Integrated Care" which wasn't an improvement. This sounded like a business arrangement instead of a clinical practice. Columbia Advanced Practice Nurse Associates (CAPNA) was the next and best choice. As with so many of our successes, it built on an accepted model: Many medical practices at Columbia were called "Associates," such as Associates in Internal Medicine. We liked the independence and cohesiveness it represented, and it built on CAP in a new and deeply organized way.

Luckily (there was always a lot of luck with us), Oxford Health Plans had recently signed a major contract with Columbia Medical Center, with preferred rates, and for Oxford, it was a great catch. So Oxford was my first stop. I met with their medical director, Ben Saferstein, and a team of administrators from the university, medical center, and hospital, and described the 2-year-old successful CAP practice. We discussed how Medicaid and Medicare already covered this level of NP care, that it was entirely legal, and that it would be discriminatory to not accept our NPs for care that was available to other populations. I doubt my moral and legal arguments made any difference, but the reality was that the Columbia physicians, their new first team, liked the idea and made the case.

The second issue that helped us was whether Oxford had sufficient primary care providers in the new Columbia network to serve that population, and who could also provide referrals to the Columbia medical specialists. Oxford wanted their network to grow and become a major insurer for patients in New York City. The problem was that there were insufficient numbers of primary care providers available for the large network of specialists and for their beneficiaries. We offered a solution.

STRATEGY TO EARN PAR REIMBURSEMENT FOR PRIMARY CARE

Carefully, and somewhat reluctantly, but bravely nevertheless, Oxford agreed it would reimburse us directly with two caveats: they would pay us a fee schedule that was lower than primary care physicians, and no, they would not list us in their directory as participating primary care providers (PCPs). This was not acceptable to us; NPs individually had been able to secure this kind of partial acceptance wherever there weren't enough primary care physicians for a given population. We didn't want to sustain that kind of inequality and differentiation. My arguments focused on three issues.

- First issue: I argued that if they paid us less, it would look like our value and competence were less. Why would they offer their beneficiaries a second-rate provider?
- Second issue: Unless they were willing to lower the premiums for patients who selected an NP as their provider, it could be argued they were billing the MD rate to patients and then giving them a cheap substitute.
- Third issue: If we weren't listed in their directory how would patients know they had an NP as an option for primary care?

Oxford agreed. In March of 1997, Saferstein sent out an internal memo to all Oxford departments titled "Nurse Practitioner System Functional Specification." He stated,

In association with Columbia Presbyterian School of Nursing, Oxford has initiated a pilot program to credential nurse practitioners as primary care providers. This pilot project is directed at extending choice of primary care providers to Oxford members. While this pilot is initiated with great enthusiasm and optimism, it is available to only a very limited number of Nurse Practitioners at present. Because it is anticipated that, over time, this program will be offered throughout the network, our information systems need to be modified to allow NP providers to operate under the same rules as other primary care providers (such as internists and family practice physicians).

What a forward-thinking and overwhelmingly supportive statement! We were delighted for the equal position Oxford gave us and for their perspective for nursing in the future. The memo went on to state that henceforth Oxford would have a three-tiered system for credentialing nursing practitioners.

1. "Columbia NPs are part of a special pilot program. They will be reimbursed at 100% of the commercial fee schedule for that region." (In actuality, Columbia NPs received a higher than regional fee schedule and instead matched the enhanced primary care fee schedule for Columbia physicians. This transpired for the same reason we had initially questioned: If reimbursement is less, doesn't this signify the provider is less qualified? And if so, can similar premium costs be fair?)

2. "Regular NPs will be paid 85% of the regular commercial fee for the region." (In actuality, this was a huge advancement for all NPs. Before the Columbia "pilot project" there was no policy on NP reimbursement, and this new policy provided new, broad recognition.)

3. "Exception" Oxford would reimburse NPs more than 85% in rural areas where physicians are scarce. If they met this requirement, they could be reimbursed at 100% of the physician fee schedule.

This policy did more than preferentially recognize Columbia NPs; it put a formal policy in place to reimburse NPs generally. This was a significant step forward for nursing.

In all the meetings we had with skeptical but thoughtful Oxford executives from their various departmental perspectives, Ben Saferstein always listened, advocated, and moved our mission successfully throughout his organization.

This was a huge success for us, and along with admitting privileges at a premier hospital, we had a model to develop a national standard recognizing highly trained NPs as equivalent to MDs. If not, why would major insurers pay us the same rate as physicians? And in Oxford's case, they paid us the same *enhanced* fee as Columbia physicians, which meant we were paid *more* than other MDs who signed up with Oxford. We were elated because we believed we would find the majority of our new patients from the Oxford enrollees.

STRATEGY TO EARN NP LISTINGS IN THE OXFORD DIRECTORY

The directory issue was less clear cut. Oxford believed that putting us in their directory was like "taking out an ad with the state Medical Society" that Oxford treats NPs like MDs. They simply didn't want to go public. Over time, they began to edge into the idea, listing us as a separate category of providers but not embedded in the physician cohort. As Oxford concluded their landmark agreement with CAPNA, they had one additional requirement: The study design would measure several parameters that Oxford's database could answer:

- Demographic information in patients
- Number of specialty referrals per year

- Number of diagnostic tests per year
- Number and length of hospitalizations
- Number of patients who changed primary care provider within Oxford
- Patient satisfaction surveys
- Reason for visit

With these data (in CAPNA and any MD practice with an Oxford population), a blunt but interesting comparison could be compiled. We agreed to submit these data, but we never heard about it again. We did not seek external funding to conduct such a study because the design was similar—but weaker—than the randomized controlled trial (RCT) which was still under way.

LOBBYING OTHER THIRD-PARTY PAYERS

With Oxford's approval in hand, I began to lobby other payers. BlueCross BlueShield was next, and they were as wary as Oxford had been, but less influenced by the Columbia physicians. Eventually I got a call from the CEO Mike Stocker, MD, telling me he was going to authorize par reimbursement for our nurse practitioners. I thanked him for his support, and he said, "I'm doing it because it's the right thing to do, but I'm not personally in support of this idea." With Oxford and BlueCross, we went to UnitedHealthcare. They were very interested and gave us full access to their practice data so that we could measure ours as well. They did not require a research evaluation, but they did ask for our business plan before agreeing to participate as an insurer offering par reimbursement and listing in their directory. We had already developed a business plan for our internal approvals, and we gave them a copy.

Par reimbursement has broadly been an easier sell than openly listing our NPs in directories. While the broader physician community wouldn't know the fee schedules we negotiated, our presence in the directory would be an open target for non-Columbia physicians.

While New York State allowed NP independent practice and full prescriptive authority, the state required that an NP must have a collaborating physician. This physician acted as backup when needed, and our NPs had always had an easy time finding those who would serve in that role. Now, with the advent of the public announcement of our new practices, many of the collaborators got cold feet. To their credit, they didn't avoid the reason for withdrawing; they feared reprisals from other MD colleagues outside Columbia who referred patients to them, and perhaps from insurers not yet in our network. Because of their concerns, several withdrew from their collaboration agreements. In the final days of these negotiations, only two or three of the original MD collaborators remained with us, and they were instrumental in our success. They were on our preferred list for our referrals.

11

•••••

External Support Gives Stability

•••••

In this same year, 1997, I joined three boards of publicly held companies, giving me a whole new group of people to help me with the school's ventures. The largest, UnitedHealthcare, became a crucial ally in our new planned private practice. The CEO, William McGuire, was another rare physician who had a view of nursing that was far beyond the parochial standing of medicine. He was a brilliant administrator, and with his wide-ranging interests (he is the world's authority on butterflies, for example) he had transformed United into a diverse set of seven businesses that would add growth, stability, and support for the unit providing health insurance. The board was a wonderful group of astute and accomplished individuals, almost all of whom had eminence in health care policy and economics.

Gentiva Health Services, a leader in homecare, also gave me entrée to another group that might be interested in advancing the nursing profession, and Cell Therapeutics, a cancer drug development company, gave me new friends on the west coast and the corporations for whom those board members worked. From these new friends, I learned how to profile our new practice as a business; United, in particular, gave us free access to one of their businesses that could help us project revenues and expenses. It was a veritable feast for those of us who had little experience or know-how in the for-profit world. Later that year I joined the board of Welch Allyn, a privately held family company that had decided to enlarge their board to represent nonfamily health care members. It was an interesting experiment. The family outnumbered the four of us new outsiders, but they were cordial and deferential, and wanted our contributions. Welch Allyn is a large, old, revered company that manufactures medical devices, from ophthalmoscopes to defibrillators. The decision-making process in a private company was different from decisions reached with boards of publicly held companies. Welch Allyn chose to become more transparent by adding independent directors; the transition was an education for me and far reaching for them. With Columbia nursing's ventures looking more like a privately held

89

company, I wanted to avoid the internal weaknesses of isolated decision making. My experience at Welch Allyn's transformation strengthened my resolve to make our processes and plans as open to controversial response as was possible.

The CAP experiment had worried the conventional medical establishment because of our added authority, coming ever closer to medical scope of practice. But we were, after all, caring for an underserved population with Medicaid as the payer, and the uproar was short lived. But now, with plans to compete for patients who had good insurance and to carry our new authority into that practice, we knew there would be cause for real alarm.

Columbia Eastside, CAPNA, and Strategic Alliances

Columbia Eastside is a practice location for Columbia physicians in midtown Manhattan at Madison Avenue and East 60th Street, just across the street from Barney's. Many specialist physicians from Columbia keep partial office hours in the building to more easily attract patients from the Upper East Side of Manhattan. A physician might have appointments 1 or 2 days at the Eastside location and appointments on other days at the medical center location. Eastside didn't have any primary care providers. The relatively new (and small) family practice department had practices close to Allen Pavilion on the Upper West Side of Manhattan. There wasn't a big demand for family practice on the upper eastside, but there was ample demand in the family-oriented neighborhood near Allen Pavilion. Specialists at Eastside, however, could benefit from having primary care in the building, to which they could refer their patients and from which they could get referrals. We suggested we could be that resource. The Medical Board and hospital at that time were in the process of making admitting privileges a permanent policy for full-time faculty NPs. They were building trust and confidence in our practice and therefore were willing to support our plan to open a practice at Columbia Eastside; once again Mike Weisfeldt led the effort.

This plan, however, did not come with hospital startup funding or salary support. We were on our own. And we knew next to nothing about billing, co-pays, financial rules, or collections from private paying patients. Fortunately, two of the major players at Columbia nursing writing the business plan had MBA degrees (Jennifer Smith and Geoff Berg), and they knew the questions to ask and where the answers could be found. In February of 1997, we submitted our business plan to the Medical Board and to Herb Pardes. We called ourselves "Columbia Advanced Practice Nurse Associates" or CAPNA. Pardes was an inspired administrator, and he knew both finance and public opinion. His guidance was instrumental in the successful development of our practice, and he became our believable and stalwart hero when all hell broke loose in the media and medical communities outside Columbia.

Although I had resisted the plea of many colleagues to show that nursing was a differentiated style of practice, the business plan for the new practice included a section on "Differentiated Primary Care Practice." Now we saw that as a market plus (more time in a visit, focused preventive care, home visits, more personalized advice, and counsel), and because we were optimistic about the randomized controlled trial (RCT) outcomes of comparability in conventional medical care, we wanted patients to see our new practice as one for enhanced primary care.

In February 1997, the RCT had enrolled 900 patients, and when complete there would be nearly 1,400 patients. No answers on comparability were yet available, and so we proposed marketing CAPNA as differentiated high-quality primary care, not as equivalent primary care.

We projected startup costs of $1.5 million for three years, with break-even reached after three years. It was all hypothetical of course since there were no other NP practices based on commercial insurance payments with which we could forecast ours. With personnel costs at $117,000 and office costs at $219,000, we projected $49,000 in revenue for year one.

Marketing and Media Training

The CEO of Bristol-Myers Squibb (BMS), Charles Heimbold, and I were members of the Commonwealth Foundation Committee on Women, and he became interested in our new practice. He knew our NPs had full prescriptive authority, but there were far more physicians than NPs who were prescribing drugs made by BMS. When I asked him for funding for CAPNA he said yes, but with a twist—one that was more valuable than dollars in our account. He proposed a gift of $2 million, which would be given to the premier medical/marketing company BMS used to develop a national advertising campaign for CAPNA; the Communications Company in Washington, DC, became our new partner. Because Heimbold was so supportive, we were fortunate to have the head of the communications company, Bob Squier, personally take the lead in media training and in designing ads. Squier had media trained several Democratic presidential candidates, so we were definitely in the hands of the master. It was a thrilling experience.

The practitioners selected for CAPNA, and others of us who would surely be contacted by the media, were given hours of careful and nuanced training in choosing the right uninflamed words to respond to the inevitable media and medical organization assaults. The medical community would be characterized as "conventional" thinking, not "outdated." Nurses were practicing new and "well-accepted" skills, not "medical care." We learned to give the message we wanted to give, which might or might not be an "answer" to the question we were asked. We described primary care as a "sophisticated specialty which can be learned by nurses as well as physicians," not an area of medicine. No one practices "independently" because patients need skills and care from a variety of professionals. It was all about being above the fray, staying calm, and avoiding confrontation. We found that we needed every bit of the training to get through the angry and threatening response to CAPNA from "conventional" medicine.

COLUMBIA EASTSIDE SPACE ISSUES

During the spring and summer of 1997, while we were getting our political training, we were also negotiating space for our new practice. Columbia Eastside was divided up among the medical departments, with each suite, or several suites, approved, and rent was assessed based on square footage. Mike Weisfeldt agreed to sublet us space in the Department of Medicine's suites. We were able to secure space for eight sessions in a week, just two shy of a full-time presence. While Weisfeldt was entirely welcoming, several of his faculty practitioners were not. Before the formal opening in the fall, we began renting space, learning the many sophisticated processes of billing, reimbursements, scheduling, referral base, new (brave) collaborating physicians, Web design, co-pay, credit card payments, and record keeping. And we once again were doing the dance of access to secure the right space. Weisfeldt's designations of sessions (half days) worked for us, but not in its initial format. Some sessions would be in a set of consult/exam rooms, and in another session we might be seeing patients in a different medical department suite. I wrote Mike that this made the faculty feel like "circuit riders" or part-time professionals. And it confused our patients, who might see an NP in one office on a Monday and in an entirely different suite for follow-up on a Friday. It was hard enough to schedule follow-up appointments with the same NP, but going to different offices added to the instability. Mike understood and consolidated our space in two contiguous sets of offices. The physicians who used those offices when we were not there were not happy. Because the sessions we were assigned were otherwise not being rented to a specific physician, those who had their assigned sessions in the morning had become accustomed to extend their hours into those unused (and unpaid for) afternoon sessions. They were entirely unwilling to vacate at the end of their allotted time, and our NPs often showed up to see their patients and the physicians refusing to leave saying, "we often run over, and we can't leave until we have finished seeing everyone." Our time frames were eventually enforced by Mike's staff, but these physicians who saw patients in the same space during other sessions refused to remove their licenses, awards, family photographs, business cards, and so on from the walls and desk, and also refused to allow us to add ours. The identifying plaque in front of the suite gave the names of the physicians, but not ours. They finally conceded we could use the exam rooms but not the consult rooms; those they said were their private professional space. We had to go back once again to Weisfeldt to get our space freed up; the physicians were homesteading in a most aggressive way. Weisfeldt solved this situation, as he had all of the other problems, by his calm, authoritative, light hand. He simply required them to do what was authorized, issuing no threats, no recriminations, but clearly there was no room for the rebels' actions to prevail.

Although we added NP identification in the consult rooms, they had to pack up and take this with them when they left. It was like setting up an office on the movie *The Sting*. Patients saw our office with NP framed licenses and certifications, and then at the end of the day they were gone. In time we had our own dedicated suite and a full-time 10 sessions a week, but in the beginning it was a little rough.

ADVENT OF MANAGED CARE: PPOs, HMOs, OUT OF NETWORK

The year 1997 was in the advent of managed care. Insurers were developing new programs with "in network" and "out of network" differing reimbursements, and some such as Health Insurance Plan (HIP), a New York City insurer, were strongly developing capitated markets, where a group of physicians got a lump sum of money to jointly manage a patient population. Other plans required a primary care physician—as gatekeeper to specialist services—even without a capitation model. These models required a strong primary care presence, with the expectation that basic inexpensive services provided by a primary care provider would limit expensive specialist care. The "gatekeeper" model, where patients could see a specialist under their plan only if referred by their primary care physician, looked like a money maker for physician groups and insurers, but few patients with choice elected to participate. The idea that free choice of provider was gone rankled many. Fee for service and more open access to specialists has become the most common mode of health insurance, but in 1997 things looked different. When we made our first blunt attempts at projecting enrollments and reimbursement, we planned that half of our patients would be in managed care plans in a gatekeeper model. The physician contracting group at Columbia was making the same assumption for their practices.

In May of 1997, *Crain's New York Business* published the news in its daily fax on health care, "The Pulse," that HIP and Group Health Insurance (GHI), large health insurers in the New York market, had begun collaborating in a new triple option insurance product. Aimed at small business, it would give enrollees a health maintenance organization (HMO), a preferred provider organization (PPO), or an out-of-network plan. The HMO (with the lowest premium) would be a staff model HMO, with all care captured within and determined by a gatekeeper; the PPO (the second least expensive), which would give beneficiaries a lower co-pay if using a physician in the PPO, and an out-of-network option were   still to be developed. In the summer, the New York City Office of Labor Relations and Health Benefits Program listed the insurance plans open to city employees. There were seven HMOs and six fee-for-service plans. Many of the HMO plans had no premium (paid entirely by the city) in order to attract beneficiaries.

MEDICAL SOCIETY OF THE STATE OF NEW YORK STRATEGIES TO CURB NP PRIMARY CARE PRACTICE

On April 25, 1997, Charles Aswad, the executive vice president of the Medical Society of the State of New York (MSSNY), sent a memo from the House of Delegates to all members of the organization focusing on two issues. One was a plan to foster affordable point-of-service plans without the requirement for primary care referrals to specialists in managed cared.

Their second issue concerned NP independence. Responding to Oxford's decision to authorize faculty NPs for direct care responsibilities, they passed a resolution that "managed organizations designate only MDs or DOs as primary care providers," and that MSSNY "continue its opposition to replacing physicians with physician extenders." A second resolution, specifically related to Oxford's agreement with Columbia Presbyterian, directed MSSNY to "seek legislation prohibiting the substitution of licensed primary care physicians with nurse practitioners."

It's not clear where such efforts were to be targeted, but in the same meeting, the MSSNY also passed a resolution that they would "strive to eliminate the lack of MD board certification as the sole reason for denying credentialing in an HMO. So, essentially they wanted NPs in a lesser position of authority than MDs, but they didn't want a requirement that those same physicians be board certified. The two resolutions viewed together raise questions about how they might argue physician superiority.

The salaries for our clinical faculty were climbing fast. By the summer of 1997, clinical salaries were above the maximum for academic salaries in their rank at the university (most clinical faculty were assistant professors). Adding 30% to a clinical salary component so that we could make a full contribution to the Columbia fringe-benefit pool was becoming untenable with the clinical sites. Most of these sites paid an add-on to MD faculty practice salaries, but not the full 30%. In part, lessening the fringe "tax" over and above a certain salary level was a fairness issue as well as an economic one. Health insurance premiums, parking premiums, and so forth didn't cost the university more for a highly paid faculty member, so why should he or she be taxed at a higher level to pay for them? The only part of the tax that reflected a difference was the amount of the fringe tax that went into an individual's retirement account. Since that amount has a maximum per year that can be tax deferred, highly paid faculty saw no benefit in having the full 30% tax taken from their high clinical salary to pay benefits if it taxed money above the amount they could invest in their retirement account.

We also knew that clinical time was most often in a nonuniversity setting, so the cost of university resources for the practice was minimal. We consulted with our medical school colleagues and adopted their tiered tax on clinical revenue; it was far less than 30% once the maximum university salary for that individual's rank was reached. This made our clinical contracts more palatable to the sites where our faculty practiced.

LOCAL MARKETING STRATEGIES

During the summer, we were gathering information about potential enrollees in CAPNA. We did a survey of businesses in the area several blocks in each direction from Madison Avenue and East 60th Street, and asked Oxford to tell us if they covered employers there. We then offered a "wellness day" free to the employers where Oxford was an insurer. We offered screening and advice on diabetes, hypertension, breast exam, weight reduction, and generally introduced them to our about-to-open practice.

In a week-by-week calendar issued in May to all the individuals involved, nine areas were noted, and "a responsible person" was designated. These nine categories were as follows:

1. Outreach to organizations where Oxford enrollees were employed
2. Fact sheets, press kits, welcome packets for patients (we included small towels for workouts, with CAPNA embroidered on them—projecting we would attract a wellness group of patients)
3. Health-related seminars—to be developed and offered to organizations
4. Methods—efficiency, scheduling practice policies
5. Money—developing methods to track budget, cash flow, expenditures, income
6. Staffing analysis—how to use faculty practitioner time when scheduling was low or nonexistent
7. Materials—medical supplies, stationary, billing access to medical center, furniture, decorating ("it should look like the dean's office")
8. Machines—dictating, computers, diagnostic equipment
9. Marketing—gala opening plus joining events such as the Columbia Health Fair and Women's Health Month

While we were juggling space issues (we were able to secure use of part of one dedicated space in the medical suite before our official opening) and attempting to do local marketing near Columbia Eastside, faculty assigned to CAPNA began to see patients. Very few appointments were scheduled during the summer, but because we were embedded in a suite where MD patients came into the same waiting area, using the same receptionist (we paid pro rata for her time), our embryonic practice looked busy. Our gala

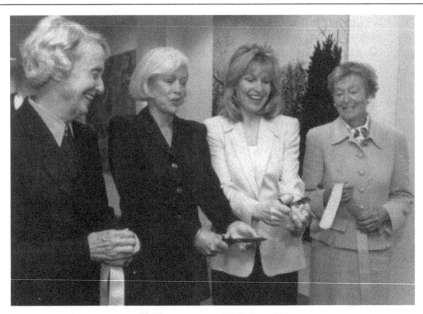

Opening of CAPNA (1997). Left to right: Dottie Simpson Dorien, president of Alumni Association; Dean Mundinger; Donna Hanover, Mayor Giuliani's wife and TV reporter; and Mary Dickey Lindsay, alumna.

● ● ● ● ●

opening was full of media, even though we had very few patients. Donna Hanover, Mayor Giuliani's wife, cut the ribbon, and we went live.

AD CAMPAIGN

The marketing we had done, which Oxford confirmed with their enrollee data, suggested that our market would primarily be individuals who worked in the area, and that this would be a young/middle-aged group, mostly women. This snapshot of potential patients was reflected in the ad campaign, which was being designed by The Communications Company, a premier firm in Washington DC. They determined that we should market to women and use the recurring theme that busy professional women didn't have time to waste when they sought medical care. The ads were smart, sophisticated, and edgy. The company also wrote a song advertisement (sung by men) with a CD cover shot of a muscled man rowing a scull. We were covering all of our bases. The audio ad would run on TV and radio, and the print ads would go in the *New York Times,* the *Wall Street Journal, New York Magazine,* and *Crain's New York Business.* Best of all, the ads would be plastered bigger than life on the sides of New York City buses. We were thrilled and giddy and ready for big time.

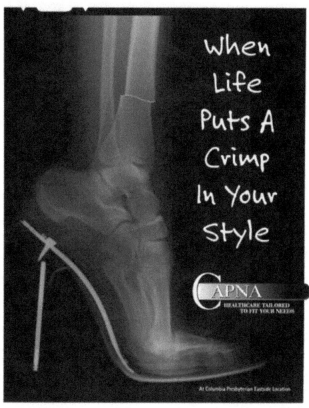

CAPNA ad that ran nationally in the New York
Times, *the* Wall Street Journal, New York
Magazine, *and on New York City buses.*

• • • • •

The first ad will always be our favorite. It is an x-ray of a woman's foot
and ankle, still wearing a stiletto heel. Clearly her ankle is broken. The tag
lines: *"When Life Puts A Cramp In Your Style* it's time for CAPNA." *"Beauty has
its rewards . . . and its price.* When pain exceeds the gain, it's time for CAPNA."

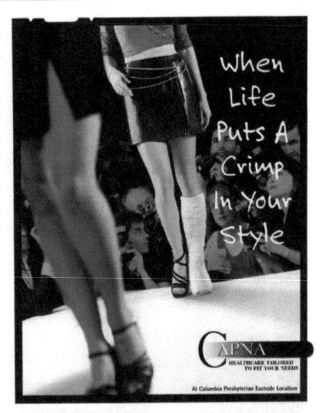

When
Life
Puts A
Crimp
In Your
Style

CAPNA

HEALTHCARE TAILORED
TO FIT YOUR NEEDS

At Columbia Presbyterian Eastside Location

*O*n the runway of life, some days you're right in style. Other days ...

So when an unexpected twist trips you up or gets you down, it's time for **CAPNA**. Columbia Advanced Practice Nurse Associates at Columbia Presbyterian Eastside location.

CAPNA is open early mornings, late evenings and on weekends. Advanced practice nurses will even make follow-up visits to your home or office.

Columbia Advanced Practice Nurses have graduate degrees in a primary care specialty, practicum experience and national certification. They can design a wellness plan to keep you fit. And they can diagnose illness, write prescriptions, admit you to the hospital, refer you to specialist physicians, and more. They're backed up by more than 300 doctors at Columbia Presbyterian Eastside location.

For more information about making **CAPNA** your primary care provider, call **212-326-5650.**

CAPNA ad that ran nationally in the New York Times, the Wall Street Journal, New York Magazine, *and on* New York City buses.

• • • • •

The next ad showed a classy model on the runway with a high-heeled sandal on one foot and a cast on the other; clearly this is the same woman. It had the same tag lines: *"When Life Puts A Cramp In Your Style"* ... "On the runway of life ... When an unexpected twist trips you up it's time for CAPNA."

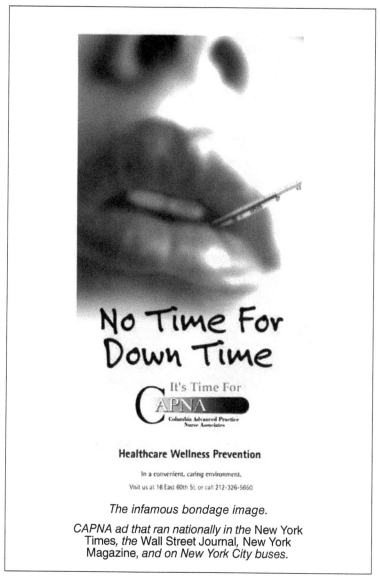

No Time For
Down Time

It's Time For

CAPNA
Columbia Advanced Practice
Nurse Associates

Healthcare Wellness Prevention

In a convenient, caring environment.
Visit us at 16 East 60th St. or call 212-326-5650

The infamous bondage image.
CAPNA ad that ran nationally in the New York
Times, *the* Wall Street Journal, New York
Magazine, *and on New York City buses.*

● ● ● ● ●

The third ad had a close-up a thermometer in the mouth of a sexy woman with the tag line "No Time for Down Time—It's time for CAPNA." We loved the ads and were thrilled at seeing buses drive through the streets of the city with our ads, and waiting with great anticipation for the next ad. We weren't sure people were watching, though, or whether we were being recognized and being considered by potential patients. We soon found out the answer was yes.

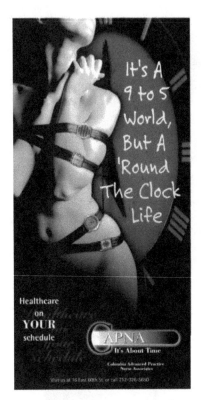

Healthcare
on
YOUR
schedule

CAPNA
It's About Time

Columbia Advanced Practice
Nurse Associates

Visit us at 16 East 60th St. or call 212-326-5660

CAPNA ad that ran nationally
in the New York Times, *the
Wall Street Journal, New York
Magazine, and on New York City
buses.*
The infamous bondage image.

• • • • •

The fourth ad was a stylized picture of the body of a woman encased in wristwatches with the tag lines *"It's A 9 To 5 World But A Round The Clock Life"*. . . "CAPNA, healthcare on YOUR schedule." The depiction was meant to show that CAPNA practitioners could see you without waiting whenever you needed care.

The day the ad first appeared on the city buses I was deluged with angry calls in my office. How DARE I portray women in bondage? They described how offensive and demeaning the ad was, and asked how a practice supposedly geared to professional women could be so insulting. I panicked and called Bob Squier. He personally arranged for a huge squadron of New York City staff to remove all the ads from the buses that same day. It was a monumental job. He never charged us for the thousands of dollars it entailed. We made no public response, but answered those who called to voice their dismay to explain what we were doing and apologize for the unintended message. It blew over quickly, but we learned yes, people were paying attention.

The other print ads continued to run in major publications. A new full-page ad ran in the *New York Times*, which showed positive quotes about CAPNA in articles published in *Crain's*, *New York Magazine*, and the *New York Times*.

After the first blitz of ads in the fall of 1997, these ads, and new ones, were placed in major publications for three years. On November 1, 2000, in the *New York Times*, for example, a quarter-page ad was published with our favorite stiletto heeled woman riding a moped and the tag line is LIFE STYLE, and a list of the ways CAPNA could diagnose and reduce risk for breast cancer.

All the ads were of an identifiable genre—young classy women who want to get what they need when they need it. And this is exactly the patient population we initially attracted. Our efforts worked to portray our practice as different in terms of attending to wellness and prevention, and personalized care that would transcend—but provide—competent diagnostic and disease treatment. The initial patients had great expectations regarding our practice, and they were not a simple healthy group. In the first week a young woman was diagnosed with breast cancer; she had previously been fearful of having a breast lump examined. Others came and had positive experiences with the thorough work-up and sent their friends. And as always, we had our loyal and dedicated New York City support group of donors and advisors, many of whom decided to give CAPNA a try and did so, and most stayed. Our male population came mostly from their significant others' recommendations. But it took nearly 2 years to enroll a significant male population. We considered adding a male NP to our group so that CAPNA wasn't so female centric, but we couldn't find the right person.

CAPNA'S COMPREHENSIVE CARE MODEL

Another group attracted to CAPNA was Medicare enrollees. In 1997, concurrent with the opening of CAPNA, the U.S. government passed a Balanced Budget Amendment (BBA) that, among other cost-saving efforts, authorized nurse practitioners as Medicare providers, to provide care in any setting.

Although NPs were rarely admitting patients to the hospital, the BBA specifically gave NPs the right to do so and be reimbursed for that care. Although Medicare sustained a fee schedule that gave NPs only 85% of the physician fee schedule, the authority for NP care was fundamentally expanded in 1997. CAPNA may have been the first group practice to operationalize this expansion. Medicare patients residing near Columbia Eastside were living in a very high-cost residential area. Many of our first Medicare enrollees already had established physician relationships, but were looking for more help with prevention and wellness approaches to help keep them fit and healthy. They had the resources to seek and follow up on this kind of comprehensive care, and they were the majority of our new patients. Again, those who did so stayed with CAPNA. Because of the high cost of living in midtown Manhattan, we had few families available for recruitment. It took a long time to recruit men, in part because we marketed to women and in part because men aren't as likely to be seeking comprehensive wellness and preventive care. In time they came because they liked the care, the approach, and the timeliness of appointments, and they valued the specialists at Columbia whom they could access through CAPNA. For the next several years we made referrals exclusively to Columbia specialists unless a patient had an existing relationship with a specialist elsewhere. But it took years before specialists referred patients to us for primary care. There are lots of reasons for this. Specialists rarely are called upon to recommend a primary care provider. Many patients go to specialists on the recommendation of their primary care provider, so no referral for primary care is needed. And although CAPNA practitioners were regularly praised for their complete and useful workups, specialists just didn't see their role as recommending patients to us. It was very frustrating because we had thought we would develop partnerships that were more than one sided. The best evidence of their support came when the specialists at Columbia Eastside agreed to list CAPNA primary care as the lead list of practitioners on the board by the receptionist when patients entered the building. This free and top billing was their mark of approval.

We struggled for years to break even, but we subsidized the practice because we believed in the model. Although primary care as a specialty was scarce throughout the country—and in New York City too—most well-insured patients had a plethora of alternatives. Anyone with a chronic illness was likely seeing a specialist who filled many of the primary care gaps as well—screening, tests, medications. Others built their own composite health care with a group of specialists—such as cardiologist, endocrinologist, surgeon, or dermatologist as needed. Well-heeled patients with a modicum of savvy were deciding on their own what physicians they wanted to see. With the collapse of HMO growth (after the flurry of activity in the 1990s), this kind of self-directed system with open access flourished. And who could say it didn't work? It was up to CAPNA to sell its brand of health care—Comprehensive Care. Part of that "sell" had to be to expanding the model beyond East 60th Street, and beyond New York. But in the late 1990s we were still focused on making this practice self-sustaining.

THE "DAY IN YOUR LIFE" PROGRAM

During our local marketing for CAPNA, in the summer before it opened, and when we identified women as our most promising population, we contacted Elsa Giardiana, a physician at Columbia who ran the Women's Health Center at Columbia Eastside. She was developing the "Day in Your Life" program, a full-day program, which included

- Medical exam
- Gynecological exam and pap smear

- CBC, SMAC, lipid profile, thyroid function exam
- Tuberculosis test, urinalysis, stool guaiac
- Oral cancer screening
- Skin cancer screening
- Vision screening

Additional services offered were

- Mammogram
- Chest x-ray
- Travel inoculations
- Nutrition counseling

Elsa invited us to participate, and it was easy to see where we could fit in as cost-effective practitioners. Here was a great opportunity to link our fledgling practice to an eminent physician in women's health care (she also had a thriving practice in cardiology and endocrinology for men as well as women). Of course we said yes. There was another valuable reason for us to participate: The center only took fee-for-service patients (better reimbursement) and had contracts with Oxford, BlueCross, and Prudential (which we already had) plus Aetna, MetLife, and Chubb. We had our eyes on Aetna. How could they not include us in par reimbursement if their peers did so? We saw participation in the center as a way to expand both our insurer base and our patient enrollees in CAPNA. Both of these efforts worked for us, but our actual participation in the center never occurred because demand for the program was too low.

CAPNA'S FINANCES

One year into CAPNA, our costs exceeded our revenues. We correctly projected a similar loss for the second year (1998–1999). We were $200,000 into the investment phase of building independent practice. This would eventually reach $1 million in investment over the first 7 years of CAPNA before the financial model began to break even. In 1990s dollars, that is a lot of money. A business assessment might say it was a very good investment for the profession of nursing, and our profession has every evidence that it is so, but the investment could only be made because Columbia nursing had the money. We never underestimated the power of our financial base. And the immeasurable value of strong and continued physician support and advocacy has no realistic price tag, but surely it outranks the $1 million we invested. The Weisfeldts, Specks, and Pardes's of the world are rare and precious, and we could not have made our mark without them. We knew that, in time, their early support would pay off. As with many wise decisions, we spent our money and political capital in the right place at the right time with the right partners. This coalescence of opportunity is rare, but it has benefited schools of nursing, the still burdened health care system, and, most of all, patients.

Expenses for the first year were less than we had projected because we had flexibility in the CAPNA NP assignments. If scheduling of patients was low, the NPs could assist with other academic work. Our projection of revenues was too high. The actual revenues ($32,663) were far less than the ($49,056) we had projected. With costs of $232,058 our first-year deficit was essentially $200,000. Our projections were built on no reliable data at all since there was none to use; the estimates were simply our hopes and wishes with a soupcon of reality. In many ways it's a wonder we even came within 70% of our wild estimate.

COLUMBIA AND PRESBYTERIAN ALLIANCE . . . FINALLY (TENTATIVE)

Presbyterian Hospital and New York Hospital merged successfully (New York-Presbyterian Hospital) under the strategic leadership of Herb Pardes and Bill Speck, working together with their Cornell/New York Hospital peers. While our own medical center remained a divided medical school and hospital, the hospital merger worked. New York-Presbyterian Hospital began its existence with the Columbia Presbyterian Medical Center and the New York-Cornell Medical Center. The merger worked because the physician leaders wanted it to and were willing to destroy the old turf boundaries. The naming was confusing, but it stuck. During these years, many hospital mergers occurred, but none combined two giants like these and none succeeded so seamlessly. It took an enormous amount of trust for the two medical schools to determine how their separate departments would work in a now single hospital system. A joint medical board was formed, with rotating chiefs, one term uptown (Presbyterian) and then a term for one downtown (New York Hospital). Although the cultures, environment, connection to their mother university, and identity patterns could not have been more different, in most cases physicians continued to admit to the hospital where they had initially practiced; there was no open competition.

For us in CAPNA, the situation was different. Cornell had not had a nursing school for decades, and nurses practicing in the way Columbia nurses did at Presbyterian was strange and alien at New York Hospital. CAPNA nurses were credentialed through the new joint departments of Medicine (and Pediatrics for those pediatric nurse practitioners practicing uptown at CAP), but the attendant admitting privileges were limited to the Presbyterian site. The joint board did not address joint admitting privileges for CAPNA and, in fact, did not do so for physicians either. Most physicians were limited in admitting to their home-base hospital site. Patients seen at Columbia Eastside were generally admitted at the Presbyterian site even though they might live and work closer to New York Hospital, which was 16 blocks south and east

The Nurse Practitioner Congratulates

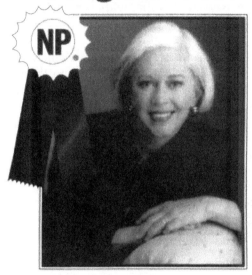

Mary O'Neil Mundinger, RN, DrPH, 1998 Nurse Practitioner of the Year.

Centennial Professor in Health Policy and Dean of the Columbia University School of Nursing, Dr. Mundinger has helped to expand the authority and autonomy of advanced practice nurses. The 1997 opening of Columbia Advanced Practice Nurse Asso- ciates (CAPNA), a new practice in Manhattan, high- lighted her role in advancing primary care. CAPNA is the nation's first primary care practice where NPs are listed by commercial insurers and reimbursed at the same rate as physicians.

Nurse Practitioner of the Year Honorable Mentions:

1. Sheila D. Behler, FNP, BSN, MSN
Family Nurse Practitioner/Director and Founder of the Center for Good Help, Detroit, Mich.

2. Judy Cohen Honig, PNP, EdD
Director of the Program in Pediatric Primary Care at Columbia University School of Nursing, New York, NY

3. Major Ronald S. Keen, FNP, MSN
Primary Care Manager of the United States Army Signal Command Fort Huachuca, Ariz.

THE ACADEMIC NURSE

Mary O. Mundinger named 1998 Nurse Practitioner of the Year

● ● ● ● ●

of the practice. If they were to go to New York Hospital, they would have their Columbia physician as a codirector of their care, while a Cornell-based physician would be the admitting medical doctor of record. But if CAPNA patients were admitted to New York Hospital, the faculty NPs could only function as consultants. This was somewhat difficult in that the NP would have to urgently find a physician in the right specialty from a department in a medical school they were not familiar with. But the NPs worked diligently to build relationships with a few Cornell physicians with whom they could fully collaborate.

Over time, and because our referrals were overwhelmingly to Columbia physicians, more of our patients were admitted to the Presbyterian site. Because the hospitals had merged, there was no reason for the hospitals to advocate which hospital site was chosen. Physicians and CAPNA NPs chose to admit patients to the one site where they had admitting privileges. The Eastside office for Columbia practitioners gave us all access to a preferred group of well-insured patients.

12

•••••

Expanding Scope and Budget Shortfall

•••••

THE SCHOOL'S 3-YEAR BUDGET PLAN (1995–1998) focused on three areas: our new Columbia Advanced Practice Nurse Associates (CAPNA) practice, research development, and enrollments. Considering how focused we were on our randomized trial establishing nurse practitioner (NP) comparability and independence in primary care, it is surprising that my budget narrative for the trustees in 1995 states that the study will "inform physicians and advanced practice nurses how to forge cost-effective collaborative teams." We had no such outcome in mind; we wanted to demonstrate we were comparable to MD practice. The wording suggests my concern that the trustees, unlike the Columbia physicians, might not support the launch of independent nurse clinicians. Trustee support of revolutionary change in an old and conservative university may have been something I worried about, but considering the support we finally achieved from them for an even more revolutionary idea 5 years later, my concerns were unnecessary.

DEVELOPING RESEARCH FUNDING

The most extensive part of the 3-year budget plan addressed our research faculty and the support we were putting in place for them. When we established the Doctor of Nursing Science (DNSc) program, the significant burden of developing and teaching new courses, candidacy and dissertation committees, determining programs and success standards, and more all fell on the shoulders of the small brigade also charged with funding their own research. It was a daunting set of responsibilities. Nonetheless, they accomplished everything expected of them, and external funding began to pour in during 1995–1996. During these 2 years we hired a part-time statistician to assist with grant submissions, and a full-time assistant professor with extensive background in evaluation research to work with faculty to develop funding submissions; we were also recruiting a senior (tenured, we hoped) faculty member to lead the doctoral program, so that our junior faculty could devote more of their time and efforts to their own research.

ESTABLISHING CAP AS MEMBER
OF THE CPPN AND ACNC

In the budget plan I noted that clinical faculty had been invited to become voting members of the Columbia Presbyterian Physicians Network (CPPN), which was the arm of the medical school charged with negotiating fees with insurers. This further solidified our standing as primary care providers. Once again, Mike Weisfeldt, president of the organization, negotiated our faculty membership. Our new Center for Advanced Practice (CAP) became a formal member of the Ambulatory Care Network Corporation (ACNC) of the hospital that same year, thanks to our other sustaining friend, Bill Speck.

ADDRESSING REDUCED ENROLLMENTS

Another major part of the budget focused on the threat of reduced enroll-ments in our master's programs. Hospitals were experiencing severe finan-cial cuts from public payers, nursing positions were being eliminated, and many smaller hospitals had closed or were acquired by bigger ones. These conditions would suggest that direct baccalaureate enrollments might suffer, but they did not. College graduates, who were our sole entry-level students, were greatly attracted to our accelerated program, and most were focused on a graduate degree in nursing, after completing the 1-year BS program and were not interested in becoming hospital staff nurses. They therefore were not deterred from applying to the Entry to Practice (ETP) program. Our mas-ter's program enrollment, however, did fall by 5% in 1995. These enrollments in advanced practice programs were all part time. As with most nursing schools, master's of science (MS) students were working full time—mostly in hospitals—and going to school part time. Hospitals had instituted many benefits for nurses when there was a shortage, including tuition assistance, which helped those nurses pursuing classes for an advanced degree. Tu-ition reimbursement by hospitals for full-time nurses was common, but was rarely available to part-time employees; therefore, this benefit mostly applied to part-time enrollment. Twelve-hour shifts—wherein a nurse could be a full-time employee while working 3 days a week—made it much easier for these nurses to schedule graduate degree coursework. With the downturn in hospital financing, tuition reimbursement disappeared or was drastically reduced, and nurses who kept their jobs had less flexibility in their sched-ules. We found ourselves at the nadir of the recurring cycle of nursing short-age and nursing surplus. In 1995 we received $2.4 million from these tuition reimbursement programs; this was exactly two thirds of all MS tuition for the year ($3.6 million). Hospitals were beginning to cut back on tuition (New York Hospital, for example, reduced its benefits from $10,000 a year to $2,000 a year as of July 1995), posting a challenge to potential students contemplating a Columbia degree, but also making full-time study more attractive: The MS degree and resulting higher level positions with higher salaries began to look like a good personal investment, one that should be accomplished quickly.

INTRODUCTION OF ON-SITE CLASSES

We developed several efforts to ameliorate this shortfall. One was to provide classes on site at a hospital if there was a large enough cohort. This we did successfully at one New York City hospital (Jacobi) for pediatric primary care. We also gave classes in blocks of time (6 hours on a Saturday, for example). While we thought this through during 1996, the cycle began moving forward again, with hospitals hurrying to meet the needs and demands of patients and benefits slowly returning. After 1 year, our enrollments were increasing once again.

Interestingly, as faculty discussed ways to transcend the hospital nursing downturn, they never suggested lowering standards for acceptance at Columbia. In part, this was because the capable students we enrolled were a joy to teach, and faculty protected this level of entry to the programs.

Even with the 5% reductions in MS enrollees in 1995, we still had a financial surplus at the end of the year. As a mark of caution, I only transferred half the surplus to the endowment, keeping half for the purpose of meeting any shortfalls in 1996. When this did not occur, these funds were transferred to the endowment the next year, along with the surplus from 1996 as well.

DNSc PROGRAM FACULTY AND STUDENT CHALLENGES

In 1996, our DNSc program admitted its third class. We had multiple challenges in this new program. Only faculty with current funding for their research were allowed to accept a doctoral student. This was one limitation. We only admitted full-time students—an entirely different requirement from the MS programs. Few nurses were willing to leave well-paying positions to fund their own full-time study; this was a new and costly expectation requirement. We believed full-time study was the most promising pattern of study to transition to a role so remarkably distinctive from clinical practice. Although practice expertise added value for a researcher (richness of potential clinical questions for study, maturity in an independent profession and more), we believed success as an investigator required a new mind set and singular immersion to develop a new career. To ameliorate these challenges, we hoped our research faculty would submit funding requests that included funding for graduate research assistantships so that doctoral students would have support. This model, of course, has been conventional and longstanding for decades in research universities. We were engaging in it for the first time, and developing researchers and research programs at the same time we were developing a doctoral program. It was a big task, and for several years we floundered on enrollments, but the faculty resources and their funding success grew rapidly. With our significant financial resources in the school, we could have simply funded doctoral students from our general revenues. But without faculty conducting research where there was a role for a doctoral student, the student would have no natural and productive mentor, no "learning lab," no role model, no growing engagement in becoming a researcher.

We had met with great success in requiring full-time study in our ETP program. These students were used to full-time study in their undergraduate years (unlike nurses who were used to part-time graduate study), and ETP students were also attracted to an accelerated program where they would become a nurse in 1 year. But this was difficult to replicate in our DNSc program, where recruits were already in high-paying nursing positions.

INNOVATIVE STRATEGIES TO SUPPORT GROWTH OF NURSE RESEARCHERS

To aid in the success of our young research faculty, we funded several members to spend time with leading nurse researchers in other universities, so they could learn how to develop scientist/mentor programs. Nurse researchers at the University of Pennsylvania (Penn) and the University of Washington in Seattle (the current top schools of nursing in the country) welcomed two of our budding researchers, one full time and one part time, at Columbia's expense. Both were supremely successful. Mary Byrne returned from the University of Washington to establish a highly funded and successful Center for Women and Children. The faculty member who participated at Penn stayed at Penn, to our dismay. Others continued to develop their skills at Columbia, working closely with physician scientists.

ADVANCED PRACTICE NURSING ROLE VISIONARY

My budget proposal for 1995 includes the observation that the role of advanced practice nurses would become the primary growth area, both in primary care in the community and acute care in hospitals. "Nursing roles will expand to substitute for many of the MD resident positions." Over time, MS full-time enrollments did grow. This was in part a reaction to the remaining low hospital reimbursement for part-time nurses enrolled in graduate programs, but there were other reasons as well. ETP graduates, most of whom had always attended school full time, were eager to continue with graduate study as full-time students. Having established "need" in the ETP program (most were no longer considered dependents of their parents), students found that continuing full time in the MS program also gave them continued eligibility for school-based financial aid, dollars that part-time students or those with a strong bank account could not access. Over time, as the ETP program grew, these graduates represented the majority of students in our MS programs. And later, with the advent of the clinical doctorate (full-time study required), ETP graduates wanted to immediately enroll in our joint MS/DNP (Doctor of Nursing Practice) program. Our evolution toward a school with only full-time enrollment was rocky but successful. We could not have transcended the interim steps without a healthy fund balance every year to pay the costs.

An important addition to our revenues was our successful submission to Columbia to receive work study funds available through the university from city and state governments for students who provided community service as a by-product of their training. Nursing students have an easily defensible position for these funds, particularly MS students who are already licensed nurses. Their unsalaried student clinical contributions would now have a financial benefit. These funds had long been available to social work students, and we benefited greatly for negotiating nurse eligibility. This was another instance of our skeptical provost providing new opportunities. We used these funds in our financial aid awards.

Common costs still made up one third of all our revenues—far greater than any databased measure could support. The big problem was that any reduction would necessarily add costs to the other health sciences schools—all of which were experiencing more financial instability than nursing. Therefore, our pleas for equity continued to fall on deaf ears (or, more honestly, on hearing that was self-protective).

SURE SIGNS OF PROGRESS

The sure progress of our increasingly complex innovations continued. Competition and full-time enrollment grew in our ETP and MS programs. The small, still struggling doctoral program began to meet its challenges by faculty sustaining our higher standards, not by eroding them. Fewer but more highly qualified enrollees gave us confidence we were on the right path. Research grants had reached $1.7 million at the beginning of the academic year, nearly all from the National Institutes of Health (NIH), which also brought in significant dollars for indirect costs, adding money to invest in our research endeavors.

In 1998, two of our innovations (CAPNA and the research doctoral program) had been launched, and we hoped we were building roots to succeed. Our finances were strong. Over $5 million was awarded for research grants. Almost $1 million was funded to expand CAPNA. Kristine Gebbie brought in eight foundation and state grants for her public health research, Joyce Anastasi was awarded nearly $1 million in an NIH grant, and Donna Gaffney had three New York State grants funded. Though dispersed in focus, productive research studies were emerging, and our NIH presence—with one star—was sustained.

During the years 1995–1999, our salary budget increased an average of 8% year and far exceeded increases in the other Columbia schools.

EMERGING PICTURE OF FINANCIAL GROWTH

Even with our NIH presence emerging, our NIH presence was small, and all federal dollars provided only 6% of total revenues and depended on one faculty member. Financial aid claimed 13% of our income on average, but the average of revenues spent on common costs stood out, even though the average of revenues spent on common costs decreased from 25% of all revenues to less than 20%. This was due to our strong growth in overall revenues each year in contrast to the other 15 Columbia schools. Nonetheless, as 1999 closed, we were still highly dependent on tuition for revenue, indeed, the percent had risen from 66% of all revenues in 1995 to 69% in 1999. The financial picture of the school was clear: We were growing, thriving, and adding new areas of growth (faculty practice, research), but we were still highly leveraged on our burgeoning enrollments. All four of the health science schools were now functioning as "tubs on our own bottom" with no subsidy from the university. We each raised all of our own money and paid the university a percentage of income for a broad and largely invisible collection of costs deemed our share. This included the downtown library, the "Crown Tax," which was a way of saying we received value for being part of Columbia.

ESTABLISHMENT OF ENDOWED CHAIRS

Following the $7 million raised for the Centennial in 1992, we made serious permanent investments in an alumni and development office in the mid to late 1990s. Jennifer Smith led broad-ranging efforts that included editing and publishing *The Academic Nurse*, our biannual journal. Four endowed chairs were established during the 1995–2000 period. The Elizabeth Standish Gill Assistant Professorship was funded in 1995 by several alumni in honor of the school's fifth leader. I knew Elizabeth Gill during the first few years of my deanship; she was an insightful, bright, imposing woman. Appropriately, Kristine Gebbie was appointed to this chair. The same year, 1995, the Professorship in Pharmaceutical and Therapeutic Research was funded by Pfizer, Sandoz, Bristol-Myers, Squibb, and Upjohn.

Elaine Larson, an infectious disease expert, was appointed to the chair. In 1996, the Helen F. Petit Professor of Clinical Nursing was established in honor of the school's seventh leader. She, like Elizabeth Gill—and all of the school's leaders except Mary Crawford—was an alumna of the school who had spent her entire career at the medical center hospital and the school. The fourth endowed chair was the Irving Chair in Oncology Nursing. This chair, fully pledged, was given by Herbert and Florence Irving, long-time active philanthropists for the Columbia University Medical Center and New York City. It will be established as part of their will.

THE ELEPHANT IN THE ROOM: TWO ALUMNI ASSOCIATIONS

In 1999, we were still awkwardly dancing around the presence of two Alumni Associations. The original was unwilling to change its mission, and the new school-based Alumni Association tried to fill the gap by focusing alumni on the needs of the school. We had an annual fund, as did the original organization, but ours was devoted entirely to financial aid for students, whereas the other organization used its funds for alumni support. The way CAPSONA (the new alumni organization, Columbia and Presbyterian School[1]) began to bring clarity to its purpose (other than the annual fund and annual meeting) was to raise money for named scholarships. This became enormously popular among alumni, who met with "their" student each year at the annual meeting. By 2010, when I left the deanship, we had 35 named endowed scholarships, each with an average value of $25,000.

During this period, we also addressed the issue of how our school should be organized. Only fully reorganized "schools" in the university can have departments. Because our school (and public health) had been departments in the medical school prior to attaining full-school status, there had been no departments but only "divisions." Our divisions were the conventional ones that mature nursing schools called departments; pediatrics, OB/GYN, medical surgical nursing. While we were still a small faculty in the late 1990s, the scope of what we were doing was greatly enlarged. We had research in public health and AIDS and advanced practice, for example, all of which transcended the scope of the previous divisions. But how should we replace those old labels? Were we big enough in any one area to merit departmental status? Did we really want to sequester faculty into a small number of departments where many might feel constrained? Most likely, many would have an interest in more than one department. So much of what we were accomplishing crossed age and specialty boundaries. Because of our success in scholarly practice, it would be counterproductive to make artificial boundaries between practice and research; between adult and pediatric care; or between acute care and primary care. Because conventional demarcations didn't reflect the diverse and multidimensional nature of our faculty efforts, we determined to forego department status for our scholarly efforts and develop something more flexible and functional.

We developed centers, which would cover broader areas of scholarly activity. We also gave faculty permission to join one or more centers, or change their membership if their interests and contributions changed.

- Perhaps the most important center developed in this era was the World Health Collaborating Center in International Advanced Practice, one of very few centers in the world approved by the World Health Organization. First established in 1995, the center focused on global research, consultation, and student experiences. Richard Garfield, the Bendixen Professor of International Nursing, and Sarah Cook, the vice dean and Dorothy Rogers Professor, have co-chaired the center since its inception. Funded research and consultations from Sweden to the Dominican Republic have been multiyear efforts of the center.
- We also established the Center for Outcomes Research, an area of inquiry we believed would be an innovative hallmark of our young research program.
- The randomized clinical trial of CAP was the anchor and name for the Center for Advanced Practice, which is concerned with the business of faculty practice contracting and practice development.
- A fourth center, the Center for Evidence-Based Practice in the Underserved, was established because of the broad faculty interest in sustaining and advancing their clinical contributions to patients with inadequate access and resources. Researchers interested in informatics contributed greatly to this center. Many faculty participated in this center, which is led by Sue Bakken, the alumni professor.
- The Center for Children and Families, led by Mary Byrne, the Stone Foundation and Elise Fish Professor in Care for the Underserved, is yet another reflection for the faculty's interest in advancing care for the populations most in need of care.
- The Center for Health Policy was the sixth configuration of this new development and attracted both practitioner and researcher participation.

The centers were not random. Each had meaning for its existing activities and values and would attract both researchers and practitioners who together represented our mission.

WHAT DID ALL THIS MEAN?

Looking back on the achievements we were making, there is one overall observation that is deeply reflective of all our work: The support and accolades came from those who benefited from our work. Yes, it took a whole lot of focus and courage for Weisfeldt, chief of medicine, and his colleagues on the Medical Board to embrace our work. But the other heroes got more than they gave. Speck got a primary care resource for his hospital, and Hubbard and Bendixen saved the nursing school (and got more than they bargained for). The university and medical center were happy to have a newly reliable contributor to financing the scope of the medical enterprise. But when we needed something that might only benefit us (common cost reduction, a new building, political clout to help resolve our alumni hegemony), help was absent. This is not new news. Only the physician support we received fell outside that conventional paradigm. Yes, we represented a new and needed primary care resource, but they could have focused their efforts on the new family practice division being formed. Instead, Family Practice was limited and constrained to support the new community hospital—serving the most underserved in our larger community. Family Practice remained a division and did not earn departmental status. It remains a stepchild in the medical center hierarchy, while the nursing practice presence has soared in acceptance and eminence.

Why would that happen? Perhaps the eminence—and egos—of Columbia physicians didn't think family practice measured up. But in supporting nursing—and not inconsequentially expecting a superior level of practice from us—they could take the primary care out of the growing complexity of Columbia medicine; enhance their national and international presence as the best of the best for referral potential; and secure nursing as their best partner for ongoing care, primary care, and sophisticated help with transplant patients and those with multiple chronic illnesses. They really did understand our value, and they saw it as enriching theirs. It was a different collaboration than they would have formed with Family Practice, a group that wanted to function like every other medical specialty. We filled a need and the physicians made a choice. To our great benefit.

Interestingly, Charles Heimbold (the Bristol-Myers CEO) made a brilliant decision when he gave us $2 million in support through his ad agency. He protected his company from a blunt broadside by the likes of the American Medical Association (AMA) by making such a gift to nurses who were moving into medical space, but he gave us far more than $2 million in value. We would not have taken such a gift and used it for advertising. It would have appeared profligate and would have raised eyebrows at the university. But a gift of advertising was quite another thing, and it was extremely valuable. I wonder if nursing leaders should take a lesson here. Sometimes it will be better strategy to ask for such a derivative gift when fundraising. Not all dollars are alike. Another benefit of this gift is the fact that with $2 million in hand we would never have been able to buy our way into the very top level of the best health care ad agency.

Three disappointments from this period of my deanship are very clear. The unfair tax for our common costs continued to fall on deaf ears, as did our pleas for a new building. Third, although our physicians' support was extraordinary, we were not receiving any referrals from them for primary care. I don't think it occurred to them that they should give as well as receive referrals. They were just too busy on the receiving end.

NOTE

1. Columbia Medical Center is the combination of the Presbyterian Hospital part of "NY Cornell Presbyterian Hospital" and the Columbia schools of medicine, dentistry, nursing and public health.

Section IV
•••••

Chasing Excellence:
2000–2005

•••••

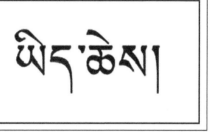

13

•••••

Turbulence and Confirmation

•••••

THIS PERIOD IN THE SCHOOL WAS ONE OF enormous accomplishment: We firmly established our new and vibrant Alumni Association, oversaw extraordinary growth of the endowment, established the first clinical doctorate in the world, and made significant progress on securing Doctor of Nursing Practice (DNP) competency standards.

While these remarkable 5 years were unfolding in our school, the context at Columbia was changing. Pardes left his Health Sciences position to become CEO of the combined New York Hospital at Cornell and Presbyterian Hospital at Columbia. This most challenging of all the nation's hospital mergers was to become the strongest and longest lasting, in no small credit to Pardes. Different cultures, geography, and history of the two venerable hospitals gave observers and pundits low expectations for success. New York Hospital was on the wealthy Eastside in midtown Manhattan, with a brilliant old-world faculty, in lovely buildings with marble halls and soaring spires overlooking Roosevelt Island and the East River, 200 miles away from the mother university in Ithaca, New York. The hospital prospered as a respected and independent medical center. The other half of this new entity, Presbyterian Hospital, was nearly 100 blocks north and some 13 diagonal blocks across Manhattan to the very border of the Bronx overlooking the Hudson River. Embedded in a bustling community of immigrant Hispanic families—more Dominicans reside there than in the Dominican Republic—the medical center was starved for space, vibrant with the same level of brilliant medical faculty, and excelling in medical research. Presbyterian Hospital—like New York Hospital—was far away from its mother university. Columbia was only 50 blocks south, but the difference in context and rhythm meant independence very similar to that held by New York Hospital. For Pardes, the differences and the big egos spelled opportunity. While he knitted the two hospitals together, adding eminence in every sphere with his charm and brilliance and hard-to-beat ideas, Columbia and the academic medical center were faltering.

A deeply troubling assault on my leadership occurred during this time and was far more painful, and the outcome more uncertain, because of the potentially diffused focus and concerns within Columbia.

The faculty I inherited in 1985 was made up of holdouts; as the school broke down, many faculty had fled to more secure positions elsewhere. Many who remained were excellent teachers for their time, but few had updated their own scholarly work; they were—understandably—mired in the past. Without the independence to chart its own future or raise its own funds, the school had been treading water in its captive position, unable to attract leadership or faculty to move forward. In our redesign of the school to be more efficient and to establish practice and research components of the faculty role, many faculty were not prepared for these new and fast-paced roles. Those who stayed experienced enormous burdens in sustaining the valued parts of their faculty contributions while stretching to learn new and challenging ones. Several faculty were studying for doctoral degrees, and many of them left because their own studies plus teaching conventional courses had been possible, but they couldn't teach, study, and also engage in the fuller faculty roles we were designing and requiring. Others wanted to stay, but unable to meet the new requirements, they left disgruntled and often bitter. The requirement for faculty practice or research was clear-cut but most contentious. A faculty committee developed these ideas, came up with a policy, voted on it, and those who chose not to comply left when the new academic year began. The research requirement was clear, although the period to succeed and comply had a longer time frame than we required finding a practice. Those who failed the new research/practice standards did not leave feeling good about either the school's new structure, or my leadership.

AFFAIR OF THE FACULTY AFFAIRS COMMITTEE!

In 2000, a faculty member who had left that year as a result of her administrative shortfalls filed a grievance about me and my leadership style to the university's Faculty Affairs Committee. Over the next 2 years, this grievance moved along its path, haltingly and often secretly, through the tortured pathways of the Faculty Affairs Committee. Instead of requiring a formal grievance and giving me an opportunity to respond, the Faculty Affairs Committee chair had covertly asked the faculty member who filed the grievance to suggest the names of other departed faculty to be interviewed to see if there was a "theme" to my administrative behavior. The committee contacted several past and current faculty—and others—and came up with a total list of eight who agreed they had been badly treated by me when they were faculty. In the end, only two of the eight faculty filed formal grievances.

In March 2001, a few months after we first learned of the Faculty Affairs investigation, the entire nursing faculty signed a letter to the president protesting that "inquiries initiated by the Committee on Faculty, Academic Freedom, and Tenure have been going on clandestinely for some nine months. Apparently, former and current professional colleagues have been solicited to come forward with reports of alleged problems with the school's administration, apart from any active grievance by a faculty member. To the best of our knowledge, only the one grievance was thoroughly investigated and resolved by the university."

When I learned of this strange and secret process late in 2000, I met with Provost Cole, President George Rupp, and vice president of Health Sciences, Gerald Fischbach to protest the workings of the committee, and to seek the names and specific grievances of those who were making statements in order to give me an opportunity to respond. I was astounded to learn that several individuals who had signed their names to the complaint, and who were protesting my administrative style, had never been faculty under my tenure as dean—some had *never* been faculty in the school. Their common status was that they were all members of our renegade Alumni Association. I couldn't believe the Faculty Affairs Committee could allow individuals with no standing to join in a faculty issue. When I raised my indignant concern, those names in the still secret report were removed.

President Rupp was advised of this issue during the last year of his presidency when he was already planning to leave the university. Provost Cole would step down from his long tenure a year later. Vice President Fischbach was brand new to his job and trying desperately to manage the medical faculty at a time of great unrest among them about space, recruitments, and the spiraling costs of staying competitive. Therefore, all three were focused on the trajectory of their own career and did not fully understand my situation.

I learned that there were a total of three grievances against me. Instead of a formal review of the three, the committee invited testimony from current and departed faculty in support of the original complainant. It felt Kafkaesque to me and alien to responsible academic practice.

During this time, I learned that in 1968, when Columbia was racked by student protests, a new university policy had been adopted to establish a process for students or faculty to have free access to discuss and deliberate—within university committee structure—any area of academic concern. There was then, and is now, a great and understandable administrative reluctance to intercede in such discussions, regardless of their merit. The fear was that any intervention would be viewed as a heavy-handed attempt to quash free speech and academic freedom. The president and provost repeatedly pledged their support of the school and its new pathways and my leadership, but they didn't put a stop to the highly questionable process of the committee. For me and the faculty, engulfed in the flames of this burning issue, it was difficult indeed.

This was a clouded backdrop and distraction from the exciting work we were doing to establish the new clinical doctorate within the university. I don't doubt the administration had good reason to step lightly on what was essentially a witch hunt meant to disable me. From the questions they asked me, and the resolution of specific grievances, I believe the Faculty Affairs Committee viewed me as having too much control, acting with impunity to set new standards and behaving imperiously. However, no academic guidelines had been breached, and all of the specific complaints about unfairness or unreasonable requirements were found to be not true.

LOOKING BACK

In the years since that time, I can see where my actions could be viewed with alarm by the Faculty Affairs Committee. We had accomplished a revolution in the school and the new faculty and able survivors were proud of our new school, but it was not a conventional academic transition. We didn't have lengthy debates about how to save the school. There wasn't time; we were on life support. That doesn't mean we didn't try to bring about the transitions in a democratic way. The research and faculty practice policies—which were the crux of departing faculty dismay—were deliberated by a faculty committee and put to a vote of faculty. Nonetheless, if one is a loser in a fair game, it is natural to look for flaws in the process. And there were flaws.

EXPECTATIONS OF FACULTY PRACTICE . . . AND PRACTICE REVENUES

Most significantly, the faculty practice contracts were confusing to new recruits. Although we had pored over the details for months to get it right, legally and professionally, this was a complex idea to new faculty. We may not have been clear enough that the time it took after being hired to secure a practice was time limited. After that, the school would not subsidize the percent of time that should have been fulfilled by practice revenues. We thought we were clear, but the idea that "good effort" without actually securing a practice was not what we required; we wanted them to have practice revenues sufficient to support their salary. We learned that nothing is more likely to cause faculty dismay and anger than seeing their paycheck cut short, even though their contract detailed such an action. We could have been better at interim follow-up with faculty in their search phase, to remind them of the time-limited subsidy. Some hoped we could have been more pro-active in helping them craft the "sell" to potential clinical employers. Faculty were not the only ones new to this fledgling idea of faculty practice; clinical sites were confused by it too. The biggest issue was why they should pay a percentage of a full-time salary—plus fringe benefits to Columbia—for a part-time clinician. We left inexperienced faculty largely responsible for making the case by themselves.

Although the challenges were great for faculty to secure practice positions and to develop research funding, most were able to do so. They succeeded against all odds, and they built the new school as we know it. Practice, in particular, brought faculty enormous satisfaction. The plan we put in place allowed them to sustain a practice component they loved, and they found that teaching wasn't an isolated second part of their new role, but was instead the stage on which they could impart their clinical acumen. The hard part was helping clinical employers understand the unique and differential value of practitioners whom we knew were constantly advancing their skills and bringing useful students (who were potential future employees) to their hospital or community-based practice. The employers who understood this opportunity saw that faculty practitioners were the most able and exciting recruits they could find for any position, and they paid the price for this excellent resource. We, in the school, however, could have done a better job helping faculty tell their story as they sought practice opportunities.

For those who succeeded—in research as well as practice—I gave them the accolades they had earned. I'm sure this was like salt in a wound for those who could not—or chose not to—do the same. In contemplating this time from any years' perspective, I could have done better. I wish I had been more tempered and experienced as an administrator facing individuals unable to perform in new and challenging standards; but I wasn't. I was chasing excellence, rewarding those who were going way out on a limb to make our new vision succeed, and I'm sure my fervent championship of the winners hurt those who did not make the cut. I know administrators who have been able to do this better, but I wasn't there yet in the late 1990s; so I paid a price, as did those who felt so poorly served by me. What remains with me as a fact of great value is that a president, just weeks from leaving the university was willing to stand up for me and for a difficult cause, that the provost, planning his own transition to a faculty position at Columbia, was willing to put his stamp of approval on my leadership in conflict with the Faculty Affairs Committee, and that the new vice president of Health Sciences, besieged by a wildly assertive medical faculty, championed my issue. I look back at a time when I initially felt vulnerable and had profound and essential support from those who—personally and professionally—had other priorities.

NEW ALUMNI ASSOCIATION COALESCES

Our new Alumni Association burst on the scene after decades of simmering concern from many alumni over the absence of an alumni group focused on supporting the school. With the old group increasingly distanced from and at variance with the school that was energized under my leadership, alumni who supported the renewal decided to form a new Alumni Association. They tried first to expand the mission of the old group without success, and when a merger was suggested that too failed. The new group wanted Columbia to anoint them as the only official Alumni Association for the school. They argued that the other alumni group was a separate 501(c)3 organization outside the Columbia structure, managed its own money, including fundraising and expenditures without university oversight, and had a mission to support alumni, not the school. The new group decided the best way to show that alumni supported them was to ask for their "vote" in writing. Dottie Dorien, the first president, was a diminutive and savvy blond, an artist and still a tri-athlete, in her 60s. She wore designer suits and had an awesome presence. Phebe Thorne, a lawyer and a judge, as well as one of our alums, was a stunning partner for Dottie in this mission. Phebe is perhaps the most glamorous, warmest, and most capable woman to ever wear a Columbia nursing pin (which she always did, attached to her judge's robe). They engaged several other smart, outspoken advocates from the alumni ranks and set out to bring about their own Columbia revolution. They sent a mailing to every alumna they could find an address for, asking them to return a postcard marked with their vote for a new Alumni Association. The cards poured in. Over 30% of reachable alumni responded. They cared. And they were willing to help. Dottie and Phebe asked me to join them in a meeting with President Rupp to gain his acknowledgment that they were the group alumni wanted to represent them. President Rupp had no idea of what these two extraordinary women planned to do at the meeting. They carried in with them a big box and unceremoniously dumped the contents of thousands of postcards on his desk. Then the discussion began.

This meeting took place early in 2000—months before the faculty affairs investigation—giving the year a distinction of two major and highly contentious nursing issues for our outgoing president to address. Who could expect courageous and strong responses in support of the school? We were still so new to our successes it would be easy for a president of a great university to say, "whoa, let's take these things slowly," and head for the door. But in both cases, President Rupp stepped into the fray and gave us his wholehearted support. In a subtle but important way, the high profile of alumni who supported the new organization—and my leadership of their school—must have had an impact on the positive outcome of the Faculty Affairs debacle that first landed in the president and provost's offices a few months later.

In early January 2000, the focus was on our new alumni organization. Rupp said he would do what he could to honor this request, and he did. With careful scrutiny from the general counsel, he sent the old group a letter stating that the university recognized only the new group as the official alumni organization. Not surprisingly, the old group refused to relinquish its status or to cease fundraising. The university was unwilling to take legal action, which could be viewed as the specter of a heavy-handed patriarchal behemoth squashing a noble band of nurses working to aid their loyal sisters. It wasn't in the cards. Nonetheless, the new group was thrilled and energized. They needed a name. And they needed a name that recognized the many older alumni who had graduated from the school when it still resided in Presbyterian Hospital. We needed their collegial—and financial—support. The name the new group adopted was almost indistinguishable from the old group; all that was dropped were two words: university and hospital. Columbia and Presbyterian School of Nursing Alumni—CAPSONA—was born. There was, of course, inevitable confusion. We were counting on time—years—to solidify the new organization. Those so uninvolved in the school for so many decades felt a certain loyalty to the old organization. They might only pay dues of $25 a year, but they loved coming to the reunion to see each other. Their loyalty was about fellowship with their former classmates, not the school. We hoped we could do both within CAPSONA, and we still hoped to find a way to merge with the old association.

Other things were happening to form the context of our work in the early 2000s. We had a new president: Lee Bollinger from the University of Michigan. A distinguished lawyer, Dr. Bollinger, while president at Michigan, successfully won the Supreme Court case testing the right of universities to apply affirmative action to increase the number of minority students. He arrived at Columbia just weeks before 9/11 and led our renewal from that day. He accomplished what Columbia presidents had desperately wanted to do for decades: moving into the adjacent acres of Harlem, an extended space that had previously boxed in the university. Bollinger doused the potential firestorm between Harlem and Columbia with a brilliant strategy of establishing important trade-offs for the community residents and commercial establishments that would be displaced as a result of the move. In the midst of this hugely political strategy, he also spent some time with us in the nursing school and supported the next step of our always eyebrow-raising proposals: the Doctor of Nursing Practice (DNP) program.

As the DNP program took shape and a new and vibrant alumni association took root, the Faculty Affairs Committee continued to hold hostage their final report; it was not clear what was going to speed up their deliberations, but it was nearly another year before they submitted a report. None of the grievances had been found to be actionable, and no academic or legal rules had been broken. Their overall assessment was that my style was an issue for those three former faculty who had left. The cloud had lifted, but it had kept the sunlight from shining on the many exciting days during that incredibly successful year.

14
•••••
The Birth of the DNP Degree
•••••

OUR MOST IMPORTANT ACCOMPLISHMENT OF the early 2000s was the development and university approval of the Doctor of Nursing Practice (DNP) degree. This occurred in the midst of a new national nursing shortage, which raised many questions about why we weren't focusing on solving that instead. Leading up to the year 2000, and into the early years of the new century, national nursing undergraduate enrollments dropped 5% a year. The deficit in nursing resources seriously impacted hospitals in particular. Johns Hopkins University announced in 2002 that it could not open its new cancer center because they couldn't find nurses to staff it. Our own medical center felt constraints as well and radically cut back units and staff available to us for clinical training. Nationally, the average age of a nurse was 44 years. Nursing was not developing new nurses to replace this aging resource, especially at the educational level needed. And even within this inadequate workforce, only 40% of nurses had a baccalaureate degree, a level of education increasingly sought by hospitals who knew these graduates had the requisite skills to care for an increasingly complex patient population.

Not only was our proposed new doctorate not focused on this issue, but our new BS program (for college graduates) Entry to Practice (ETP) students were not interested in filling this gap. They valued their hospital bedside experiences but did not view that career as their choice.

In 2002, the argument for a DNP went against the grain of conservative thinkers, who thought we should be meeting the national need for hospital nurses, not developing elite roles. We believed otherwise. Columbia University resources had always been devoted to the highest levels of achievement in any calling. In medicine, Columbia's goal was to train physicians in the most complex and emerging specialties. The same cutting edge focus was true in the other professional schools as well. It may be that our struggle was amplified by Columbia nursing's late entry to graduate study, and the fact that the majority of members in our profession didn't even have a baccalaureate degree. Many in the larger university viewed nursing as a homogeneous profession, which we have never been. We had a challenge to convince our Columbia colleagues (outside of medicine, who had helped us build the program) that a clinical doctorate was reasonable, had merit, is where Columbia should invest its nursing resources, and was a safe bet for the university to publicly support and offer to the public.

As we began to seek approval of the new degree within the university approval process, many at Columbia didn't even know the university had a school of nursing. Embedded in the scholarly life of Columbia's main campus, faculty had an understanding that physicians and dentists and public health professionals were earning their graduate degrees uptown, but nursing was an invisible entity. Because our academic standing was so long in developing, we weren't even known for conventional contributions to academic health center research. And here we were, showing our heads for the first time in the senate of a conservative bastion of the Ivy League, and asking for approval to be recognized for a totally new doctoral-level education—in clinical care. We didn't even have our first *research doctoral graduate* yet. No one knew what a clinical doctorate in our profession meant. Hospital nurses? Well yes, maybe, but different from what one thinks of as dedicated, smart nurses at the patient's bedside who take their orders from "real" doctors. We had to make the case in the context of extreme ignorance of some faculty senators, one of whom famously asked me at a formal hearing, "If you give them a doctoral degree, who will carry the bedpans?" Others were more knowledgeable about our renewal and contributions, but were wary of how such a new and untested invention in Columbia was viewed and how this would fit in a legacy for excellence, which had been established conservatively at the university. One administrator asked, "How do we know other universities like Columbia will adopt this degree? What if only lesser colleges come on board? How will Columbia look then?" They were looking for some evidence that the medical community (at home and nationally) would view this revolutionary idea positively, and that our most prestigious academic nursing colleagues would join us in this endeavor.

As we dealt with Columbia's understandably conservative nature and the skeptical medical and nursing leaders across the country, we did two things that helped our cause. In the late 1990s, we developed a Board of Visitors and made a big effort to publish our views and research on the DNP program. The Board of Visitors was designed to give influential advice and support to our new initiatives. Members were recruited mainly from our alumni leadership who had bravely established the new alumni association, and from health policy leaders in the city and from afar. Karen Katen, senior vice president at Pfizer, Phil Nudelman, CEO of the Hope Heart Institute in Seattle, Elizabeth McCormack, of the Rockefeller Brothers Fund, and Phyllis Farley, a major New York City philanthropist, all joined forces with us to provide the university—the trustees more than the hunkered down senate— with their support. The board members added far more than support for our ideas: They challenged us in the content and understandability of what we were doing. With our discussion in the school under constant tweaking, bursting with "why not" questions, we were growing daily in our understanding of how to develop our new doctorate, the competencies necessary, the skills to be tested. We would emerge every month or so from what were breathtaking advancements and place them de novo in front of our board for their expected adulation. Mostly they wanted to be supportive, but they were often confused by our ideas. We knew how we had arrived at the goals we were promoting, but they hadn't been with us in the step-by-step deliberations to get there. We realized our exciting and collegial plans needed far more explaining. We took another step on a very conventional path: We published our ideas in all the major nursing publications, focusing on our innovations, our influential partnerships with AACN, and the remarkable job the organization was doing to recognize plans for this new degree.

DNP FOUNDATIONS IN EXPERIENCE AND EXPERIMENTATION

As with every major breakthrough, our DNP plan was rooted in years of experience and experimentation. Most master's degrees in advanced practice had expanded to include a scope of skills and competencies that merited doctoral degrees in other professions. Those with a BS in nursing and an MS in advanced practice had spent more years learning their profession than those in similar years of training who earned the title of doctor: ETP students entered nursing school, as did medical students, after 4 years of preprofessional undergraduate education. After an additional 60 credits to earn a BS in nursing and 60 credits in MS education, they had 120 credits of graduate work (as did medical graduates) with no doctoral title. In the health care world, *we were the only profession without a doctorate in our core competency of practice. We had given that away when we developed MS degrees instead.* This gap hurt us, especially in the broad view of nursing as a group under the direction of physicians. This limited professional recognition, but also limited authority to give care independently and to receive direct payment for those services. Titles—and degrees—matter.

At Columbia, we were intent on formalizing the practice advancements our Center for Advanced Practice (CAP) clinicians had learned when they participated in the randomized trial. Why should nurses everywhere have to develop their own ad hoc advanced training to do what CAP nurses had shown could be done? Why not institutionalize the learning of those skills and knowledge, put the right title on it, and work toward national adoption? We had been further encouraged about our model as the Columbia Advanced Practice Nurse Associates (CAPNA) experiment succeeded. This proved that nurses with these highly developed new skills were acceptable to patients with commercial insurance who could choose any physician they wanted—and many chose us: This was a marketable idea as well as a professionally satisfying one.

THE EMERGING DIVIDE BETWEEN THE CLINICAL
AND NONCLINICAL DNP

Other schools were also contemplating a new doctoral degree for nurses. The University of Kentucky formulated a plan and called it the Doctor of Nursing Practice. But it looked nothing like our DNP program.

Kentucky viewed "practice" as advanced nursing actions and decisions, but not necessarily clinical ones. They crafted a curriculum that gave graduates the skills to design, manage, and evaluate complex systems in nursing. This is essentially a sophisticated management role, one that Kentucky— and others—call leadership training. While valuable as an option to a PhD research degree, it is not clinical care at the doctoral level. The nonclinical practice doctorate rests on the belief that MS-level clinical practice plus the ability to perform sophisticated systems and management skills, preferably in a clinical setting, somehow equals a doctoral degree in nursing practice. One has to take another step off the path, however, to rescue the validity of the nonclinical DNP. One has to believe that "practice" encompasses the role of a nurse in any professional endeavor and is not limited to clinical care.

These are awkward arguments indeed. Many alternative doctoral titles could have been used for a sophisticated nurse manager who had achieved an MS degree in clinical practice along the way. A legitimate doctoral title for these nurse system managers/leaders could have been selected that didn't end up redefining the exquisite and fundamental practice component of nursing. Is a physician engaged in "medical practice" as CEO of an insurance company? Is a dentist engaged in "dental practice" while managing a community wellness program? There was no reason nursing chose to be an outlier. Except for one.

Nurses have long been angry and frustrated that their clinical practice is viewed as a subset of, and beholden to, medicine. Nursing Practice and its eminence was a burning issue in the 1990s (and perhaps every decade since Florence Nightingale). A few education doctoral degrees were still being offered, but they were largely an unattractive choice for nurses who felt limited by an education degree, and which was not representative of nursing's core contribution, its practice. PhDs for nurses, in nursing or in other disciplines, were strong degrees, and those with PhDs found their stature in research and academia was respected and secure. But not all nurses wanted to be researchers, although many wanted to earn a similar and respected title— doctor—to represent what they had achieved in their professional careers. In searching for the right title, they chose "practice," which had heft and significance.

It's not surprising then that the focus of this new DNP degree would be more than clinical. It wasn't to be an education or research degree, but rather a degree that would recognize the differentiated high-level nursing careers they had chosen. However, those most vigorously pursuing the idea of a new nursing doctorate weren't really practicing nurses anymore; they were administrators and educators. They wanted the imprimatur of "doctor" in their new nonclinical, nonresearch careers. So the long unfilled gap for a doctoral degree specific to our profession—the DNP—was adopted by those who could see the power of the title, but who were not planning to prepare for a new and higher level of clinical care.

COLUMBIA'S VISION: GROUNDING IN DOCTORAL-LEVEL NURSING PRACTICE

This tortured rationale nearly drove us crazy at Columbia. We agreed our profession needed a doctorate that recognized practicing nurses at the doctoral level. We just couldn't believe that our own innovative, long, and carefully evaluated program with the goal of recognizing doctoral-level nurse clinicians, was being hijacked by well-meaning academics who had another goal, one that opened the door for worsening the public's understanding of nursing, instead of clarifying and advancing it. Not only was the DNP title highly appealing to those who wanted a new degree, but there was another reason a high level of clinical acumen was not included in most of the new DNP degrees. Faculty in schools contemplating a new doctoral degree had not developed doctoral-level clinical practice, as we had done over a 10-year period. If they couldn't practice at that level, how could they fully understand it, and, most fundamentally, how could they teach it?

Many of the nursing faculty who were developing the new degree knew better, (our work on new doctoral-level clinical skills had been detailed and published for years), but they adopted the stance that those with an MS degree in advanced practice represented the highest level of clinical nursing care. Therefore, a practice doctorate would simply build the infrastructure components around the skills achieved in MS degrees. This opinion naturally attracted strong and vocal support from advanced practiced nurses with master's degrees. Their support strengthened the resolve of faculties who wanted a DNP degree, but who had no resources or knowledge to develop doctoral-level clinical content. How easy it was to simply accept MS-level clinical skills as the standard, add doctoral-level courses in nonclinical areas, combine the two, and end with a doctoral degree in practice. These advocates argued that our CAP and CAPNA levels of practice were widely practiced by MS prepared nurses. They believed that nothing more was needed in the clinical realm to earn a DNP and that a DNP graduate should only need to achieve additional skills in the administration, system management, and technology support for advanced clinical care. Epidemiology, biostatistics, and "clinical experiences," which consisted of managing or evaluating care, were somehow equated with achieving a higher level of practice, nursing practice. It still drives us crazy.

THE UNBRIDLED GROWTH OF THE DNP

The nonclinical DNP took off unbridled and with great diversity from school to school. This unstandardized nonclinical nonresearch doctorate was quickly developed by dozens of schools and was aided by the ease of providing instruction. No clinical sites for students were needed—always a chore—and no faculty with the new advanced clinical skills demonstrated by the Columbia clinicians was needed. Existing nurse faculty were sufficient. Support courses could be found on the web (or in schools of public health or business on their own campuses) and adopted by bright energetic nursing faculty. Courses in leadership and systems management were long a part of nursing Administration and could be codified or adopted as doctoral courses. No time-consuming one-on-one carefully mentored research training was required.

Except for the core difference in clinical care education, all DNP programs require similar courses. Some have established PhD-like DNP programs, which are essentially focused on research, but with less emphasis on becoming independent investigators. Valued skills in collecting useful data, helping a PhD investigator develop credible outcomes measurements in studying evidence-based care, and many other collaborative skills add greatly to the nursing research community. DNP graduates from these programs possess an amalgam of MS-level clinical skills and research support skills. Their clinical acumen adds enormous value to a research design that aims to study clinical outcomes or cost-effective care. This clinician viewpoint continues to assist in the development of policy yielded from such studies. But these graduates are neither doctoral-level clinicians nor independent researchers. Valuable indeed, but doctoral level? It seems to me that a doctoral degree represents the top of the line in a defined area of expertise. DNP graduates who add research skills to their MS-level practice are neither the highest level clinicians nor the highest level researchers. They are a wonderfully rich contribution to nursing, but is this a doctoral achievement?

At Columbia, we tried to figure out where we should go in this environment. DNP programs without doctoral-level clinical practice were flourishing. Understandably, very few faculties were emulating ours. We had taken 10 years, millions of dollars, a devoted courageous focus by faculty already in a formal faculty practice model, and a medical school and hospital that invited and supported this advancement to end up with our DNP program. For those faculties contemplating a clinical DNP program, how could we at Columbia help make this happen?

We had several ideas.

- We could free up some *circuit riders* from our DNP level faculty, and send them to other leading schools of nursing to introduce and teach the new skills and work with the nursing and medical faculties there to take it on themselves.

- We could publish some kind of primer.
- We could develop a group of influential nursing deans and help them put programs together.
- We could try to get major foundation funding for a collaborative, capturing new recruits.
- And, most importantly, as we acknowledged it would be folly to think we could abolish all the nonclinical DNPs, we could find a way to distinguish the clinical DNP programs from those which were not.

Eventually, we tried all of these approaches. Some were very successful, and others were not.

As we were involved in this rather chaotic "let all the flowers bloom" nursing environment in 2001, we at Columbia decided to go full speed ahead in evidencing the components of a clinical program. If we weren't going to be the *only* DNP model, we could then at least be the *first*. President Rupp had left the university to become head of the International Rescue Fund, a mission close to his heart. He has passionately and successfully led the fund, folding his lanky frame into coach seats, flying across the world for over a decade of great progress. Lee Bollinger arrived as our new president as we were preparing our DNP proposal for university approval. At the University of Michigan, where he served as president, nursing had a long and distinguished reputation for research. Their reputation in advanced practice was less visible and less a part of the school's primary mission. Bollinger understood and respected nurse researchers. We asked him to meet with us to discuss our proposed clinical doctorate, and he came up to the medical center to hear our story. The faculty who were accomplished and practicing with DNP-level skills were articulate and knowledgeable. Not surprisingly, many had earned research degrees before re-committing themselves to clinical practice. They had the unenviable task of convincing our new president that Columbia should approve this new level of practice (always difficult to explain to non-nurses since we tend to have our own self-defeating language), but to also assuage any worries he might have that Columbia might stand alone with this new degree in the future, or worse that only lesser schools would follow our lead. I was proud of the clinicians' presentation, but it was our researchers who carried the day.

Although new to a research focus, Columbia nursing faculty had made remarkable progress in achieving funding for their studies. Kristine Gebbie had been head of state health departments in both Washington and Oregon and was President Clinton's appointee as the first AIDS czar before joining our faculty. Her generative contributions in developing the nation's public health workforce were funded by all the major health foundations. Even with this one of our major researchers funded outside the National Institutes of Health (NIH) stream of priorities, we had a breathtakingly successful

NIH funding record. As a small faculty we couldn't achieve the most dollars of NIH funding per year, but we *could* show that our faculty had an outstanding record per faculty member. Our national ranking as a nursing school rose from 59th to 20th from 1998 until 2003. We can only reasonably expect a higher standing if we triple or quadruple the number of researchers on our faculty—an accomplishment depending primarily on space (a new building!). But our small band of researchers was the best in the land. And we even had some important metrics to prove it. In 2000, our per capita NIH funding reached number one in the nation. And this wasn't simply a quirk of our small size—our closest competitors on a per capita basis were also the most highly ranked NIH schools in the country. In 2001, we slipped to number two in per capita funding as we hired two junior researchers who were not yet funded, but in 2002, we reached number one status again. Here are our colleagues in the top seven (per capita) in 2002:

	NUMBER OF RESEARCH FACULTY	DOLLARS PER CAPITA
Columbia University	12	136,289
University of Pennsylvania	44	130,872
University of Pittsburgh	44	116,750
University of Illinois	75	109,017
University of California at San Francisco	103	103,527
University of California at Los Angeles	31	99,159
Yale University	30	97,007

We didn't let this achievement go unknown to our new president (Michigan wasn't in the running for our new way of ranking faculty research). Importantly, these extremely successful NIH researchers at Columbia were not simply focusing on their nursing initiatives. Each of the (then) three tenured professors at the top of our research success also held joint appointments in other Columbia schools: Sue Bakken in the Department of Informatics in the medical school, Kris Gebbie and Elaine Larson in the School of Public Health. Whereas our eminent clinicians were visibly engaged in the medical school where they held appointments for practice, it was not as well known that our research faculty was equally engaged in interprofessional work. This, too, was not lost on President Bollinger. Given the high regard our researchers held at NIH, foundations, and our Schools of Medicine and Public Health, and because research is a strong and essential part of Columbia University, Bakken and Larson and Gebbie, as well as younger and productive researchers, helped our pioneering high-level clinicians convince our new president he should cast his lot with us. Our strong financial position, with millions of dollars available for the successful roll-out of a new degree, also strengthened our position. When I walked out with Bollinger after the meeting, he said, "I am very impressed with your faculty. You have my support for the degree."

THE RACE TO THE FIRST DNP GRADUATE

We began the race to graduate the first DNP student in the world. But first we had to get the degree approved. As that process went through its glacial pathway, we received approval from the provost to engage in a highly unconventional plan. We proposed to fully develop all the DNP courses, ask faculty who were not candidates for the degree to teach them, and conduct the DNP program solely for our faculty before the university approval was achieved. The provost agreed. I pledged that we would not use the opportunity without faculty understanding that their enrollment in this program might end up without the university granting the degree. They were willing to take the chance, and nearly every faculty member in practice—not just the CAP and CAPNA pioneers—and our star NIH researcher, Joyce Anastasi, enrolled in the program.

We couldn't simply anoint those who were already practicing in the new higher level of care; they had to participate in all the courses. But some of them were experts in their field, with knowledge all DNPs were required to possess. We therefore, gave them assignments for specific lectures in courses, but no "students" were course directors, nor did they evaluate any student's work. Again, our research faculty came through for the DNP, assuming course director and lecture responsibilities for all the new courses. Many collaborated with colleagues in the Schools of Business and Public Health to formulate the new courses. We asked our physician colleagues who had been instrumental in the CAP and CAPNA practices to teach the formal courses on sophisticated diagnostic skills, emergency room and hospital management, in-depth medical knowledge in the major categories of interventions (cardiac, respiratory, and gastrointestinal diseases), how to follow up on complicated advice from specialists, and more. Not a single physician said no. We told them this was a one-time-only request until we had our own DNP graduates. After teaching our faculty, several physicians told me they really enjoyed the experience and would like to do it again. While this was an incredibly challenging time for all of us, it was deeply satisfying to be doing something so exciting together. One faculty member, Jennifer Smith, wanted to be one of these groundbreaking first DNP graduates and went on to fulfill the MS requisite for advanced practice concurrently while earning the DNP. She already had her BS in nursing, as well as an MBA and MPH (Master of Public Health)—but this new opportunity was simply too special to let it go by.

The faculty DNP program took place evenings and weekends. No one gave up their other faculty responsibilities. Lunchtime was no longer given to a collegial hour and break from work: Faculty congregated in the student skills lab to practice on each other. Lunch was something you did on the run at another time. Regular dinner hours disappeared too, as our courses often ran during the late afternoon and evening.

The courses were given over two semesters and a January term. Faculty scheduled their clinical experiences on hours and days when they were not scheduled to teach. The degree requirements included having an article published, or in press, in a peer-reviewed journal. The article had to have clear relevance to the essential competencies for the DNP degree. They also had to write 15 case studies in a new and complex format, which in the aggregate gave evidence of their having mastered all of the essential competencies of the program. The case studies were more complete and exacting than many PhD dissertations; we did this on purpose. We didn't want the DNP to be a lower-level achievement. Publishing in a peer-reviewed journal, however, was the most difficult part of the process for many of the DNP candidates. They all wrote stunningly engaging and knowledgeable case studies, but most had never published their work before. Several grasped their acceptance letter from journals with more glee and sense of achievement than when they handed in the tomes they developed with their case studies.

We just about exhausted them with our above-all-reproach faculty program. But not in vain; the university approved the program just days before the first university degrees were offered in early 2005. Jan Smolowitz, DNP, took her place as the first graduate of a DNP program in the world. By May, we had 19 more, and everyone—faculty and faculty students—celebrated the landmark achievement for themselves, for their colleagues who taught them, and for their school. It was a magnificent way to mark our 20-year renewal in the nursing school.

Before we began the faculty program, we had to finalize the courses and clinical outcome measurements. This was not easy. The CAP and CAPNA cohorts were all educated in primary care; they were adult, pediatric, or family nurse practitioners. The care they provided, however, was more than primary care. We relied on accepted historical definitions of primary care to make this distinction: first contact, continuing care, in the context of family and community. Primary care in medicine had evolved from the general practitioner who saw patients in his office, the hospital, and often in the patient's home to an office-based clinician who was the conductor of a growing orchestra of specialists for his patients, providing basic care for less urgent conditions, and caring more and more for an essentially healthy population, and those with chronic illness. Most could no longer offer the time to follow their patients who were in the hospital under a specialist's care. Increasingly, primary care became an office-based practice, and one in which nurse practitioners worked closely—and sometimes indistinguishably—with physicians. As primary care became filled more with wellness and chronic illness care, physicians who were educated for a much broader and fast-paced career began to leave primary care, or never choose it to start with.

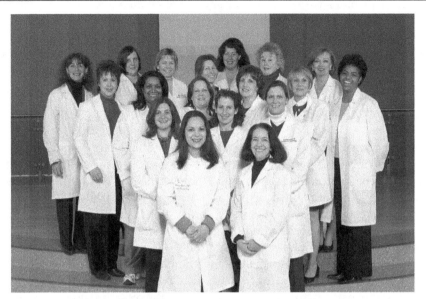

First DNP graduates from Columbia University School of Nursing (2005).

● ● ● ● ●

As physicians left primary care, nurse practitioners (NPs) moved in. And the specialty changed dramatically—not because NPs took over, but because the scope of patient needs became more complex. With medical advancements came longer, but more vulnerable, life spans. Chronic illness wasn't as simple to manage as before, with more unstable conditions, and frailer surviving patients, who had more comorbidity. There was more a clinician could do, and more and more sick patients to do it for. A hospitalization could no longer be fully managed by a specialist for one condition when the patient had several other specialists. And even without the radical changes in medicine and survivability, people were changing in what they demanded and expected from the health care system. The Internet and proliferating health websites turned patients from consumers to quasi-experts. And with the cascade of promising new medical therapies, cost of care skyrocketed, as did the need for more specialists to provide this sophisticated care. Just as medical specialties expanded, so did the role of primary care. It was no longer sufficient to provide primary or first access to health care, or even the continuing source of care for chronic illness and newly diagnosed conditions. Caring for those needing office-based care and referring to the growing army of specialists for complex interventions were not enough. Comprehensive care encompasses primary care: first access for patients with new symptoms, new disease, or advice and interventions to prevent illness or disability. This aspect of primary care is essential and more challenging as more can be done, and patients can learn to do more to protect their health. The role of specialist has grown as the ways to treat illness have grown; hospitals are no longer places to recover as well as to undergo care not possible in an outpatient setting—hospitals have essentially become intensive care units (ICUs).

COMPREHENSIVE CARE: THE NEW PRIMARY CARE

The new primary care—comprehensive care—requires professional skills in every setting where patients receive care: making hospital visits, ER evaluations, phone (or e-mail) assessments, legal, regulatory, and reimbursement attentiveness, negotiation skills with patients to formulate what promises the best outcome for the patient. Conventional primary care often provided some or all of these services, and the general practitioner of the 1940s surely is an early but less sophisticated example. Today, patients are more likely to have a constellation of specialists they manage themselves. The clinician who replaces the disappearing primary care professional has to be more attuned to this pattern, to provide the nexus for the often lost coordination of care, making necessary global assessments—providing care that recognizes and fills the gaps in the disparate medical needs of patients. Contributing to an ER evaluation or hospital plan of care is crucial for patients who have health issues that transcend the discrete situation currently being treated. Underlying diabetes and neurological and cardiac illnesses may not be immediately evident in an emergency situation, but can compromise the outcome of care provided. A comprehensive care clinician not only knows this critical background information but has the skills and authority to participate in emergency care, can intervene on behalf of the families' needs during such an encounter, and can better understand a patient's postemergency need for care.

In a more conventional, historical pattern, nurse practitioners became highly productive clinicians in primary care. They worked in tandem with physicians, and since 1972, have had Medicaid reimbursement for sole primary care practices. In each of these environments, however, the job expectations were usually limited to office-based care, Monday through Friday. Being on call by phone or e-mail was often part of the responsibilities. But the broader cross-site responsibilities, and a more sophisticated understanding of the treatment of illness and disease, have only become necessary components of comprehensive care in the past two decades. As physicians increasingly exit primary care roles, leaving the field much more complex, it is ripe for nurses with advanced education to make this specialty their own.

Our CAP and CAPNA faculty were highly intelligent and seasoned in primary care. In preparing for the randomized trial, additional skills were necessary for the CAP clinicians; as they then prepared for CAPNA, it became evident that even more skills were needed. Commercial insurers and private patients had even more requirements and demands than in our comprehensive practice with Medicaid patients. The learning was incremental, often informal, and opportunistic. Figuring out how we could deduce a doctoral curriculum from our experiences and evaluations was daunting. Did we start with what our experienced faculty already knew when they prepared for more sophisticated, cross-site medical care in CAP? Or should we develop a curriculum for a newly minted MS graduate? How could we devise a comprehensive set of courses and clinical experiences to develop graduates who would be ready to practice as full-fledged comprehensive care clinicians?

Distinguishing comprehensive care—doctoral-level practice—from primary care as it had conventionally been practiced by MS educated nurses was a compelling goal. We believed that a clear and detailed curriculum and differential competencies would give us a strong beginning to do so. We also believed this would help distinguish clinical from nonclinical DNP programs. If we could show a measurable difference between MS and DNP clinical acumen, we could show the difference between the clinical and nonclinical DNP programs. An important ally during this process was the American Association of Colleges of Nursing (AACN).

WHAT DEGREE SHOULD IT BE: DNP OR DCP?

As schools across the country developed DNP programs, AACN president Polly Bednash, and her knowledgeable staff, worked valiantly to establish appropriate standards for the new degree without imposing specifically detailed content of the curriculum. There was remarkable agreement among schools on the nonpractice components of the degree. These encompassed the ones we had developed. A broader definition of practice was adopted. This approach sanctioned clinical practice, research practice (supportive skills in research, not PhD standards that have never been profession-specific), systems management practice, and the vague term *leadership practice*. It was up to each school to determine the practice component of their degree. This outcome was not a surprise, but nonetheless a disappointment for us, which reflected the belief that our model was not going to be able to compete with easier to launch programs. We also felt that a long sought and important goal for nursing—independent clinical practice—would not be a clear competency held by all DNP graduates. In fact, a great majority of DNP graduates would lack those skills. Most of all we felt a crucial opportunity had been lost for our profession, by recognizing these highly skilled clinicians with the same degree as systems managers. If we were ever to convince the public that we were a fully standalone clinical profession (leading to direct reimbursement from all payers, more enticing careers, and more recognition), this botched use of the title only hurt that progress.

Of course, we could have demurred in joining the burgeoning number of DNP programs. We could have chosen a distinctive title all for ourselves (and the other small number of schools who were truly teaching advanced clinical care). We considered Doctor of Clinical Practice (DCP). It had a nice ring to it. DCP sounded weighty enough. But we had reasons not to go that route. Perhaps most instrumental was our thinking that we could persuade schools to work toward clinical practice—the way we meant it—in their DNP degrees. We thought that as the clinical programs were established, the systems management and leadership degrees might pale in attractiveness to potential students. These programs might be right for nurses already set in their management careers and in need of a doctorate to hold peer status in their work environments, but nurses in the future might not aspire to management degrees if they would attain eminence in practice. This is what had spelled death for EdD and DNSc degrees, popular at their inception but outpaced by the stronger PhD. We hoped the same would happen in regard to the nonclinical DNP programs. We saw in our own innovative ETP program for college graduates (a program now extant in universities across the country) that students were very clear about pursuing doctoral education early in their careers, and they wanted overwhelmingly to be expert and independent clinicians or fully trained researchers. None were aspiring to an administrative or systems management career. We were betting on the evolution of how nurses would select a doctoral program in the future. We were betting our kind of DNP program would thrive.

But, you might argue, we could have done that more easily and quickly by choosing a title other than DNP. We contemplated the outcome of such a move. If we did so, we would be seen as outliers in a profession that highly values collegiality and acceptance within its mindboggling different levels of education. We would simply be adding a new one and would have the added burden of differentiating ourselves from DNP programs, which professed to be clinical because they incorporated MS proficiency. A public that has to understand diploma, AS, BS, MA, MS, EdD, PhD, and DNSc nurses, would then have two new doctoral degrees to try to untangle. This was not for us.

And perhaps most persuasively, we wanted to be within the tent where DNP determinations were being made. We wanted to have time and access to sell our product. AACN was doing a credible job in defining nonresearch doctorates—the broader challenge for DNP degrees. We would stay in the fold, counting on more influence to advance the DNP clinical degree. We wanted to be a part of that important process. And, not insignificantly, we already were far along the process to gain approval for the degree at Columbia. An early concern of Columbia leaders had been whether we were initiating a new and vibrant degree that other universities would adopt, or whether we were going to be an outlier. Changing the degree title partway down the path of approval gave us pause as to how Columbia would view this. We decided to stay in and find other ways to distinguish the unique clinical skills of our graduates and to work toward common standards in the future for "practice" in the DNP degree.

15
• • • • •

Should We Keep the DNP Title?
• • • • •

IN 2000 WE WERE RUNNING fast to formalize and advance our new level of practice. Columbia physicians had given Columbia nurses the opportunity and generous support to establish this advanced role, and now we had to name it and describe it in a way that others could achieve the same competencies. Our insular programs in clinical practice from 1986 until 2000 had burst upon the broader professional horizons with the *Journal of the American Medical Association (JAMA)* publication in January 2000 comparing physicians with nurses who had been trained to conduct the same medical practice in primary care. The comparability was powerful, but the nurse training to achieve that comparability had been individualized for our seasoned faculty group and had been rather informal. Moreover, the transfer of knowledge and patterns of communication and practice were often accomplished through one-on-one partnerships with a physician. Our challenge was to deduce the elements of science and skill that needed to be taught in order to replicate the competencies our practitioners had achieved. These competencies would then be the basis of the curriculum.

We struggled to name the differentiated skills of this new level of practice. A critical piece was the ability to give care across settings to the same patients—not site-specific care but cross-site care. We also knew there was a profoundly different accountability that was established with this kind of continuity of care, accountability that was more powerful and more exquisitely attuned to fostering the health of every patient entrusted to these practitioners. No hand-offs to specialists or to the emergency room (ER). Specialist referrals and ER visits were still necessary, but these were now two-way encounters ensuring that specialist responses or ER reports were shared with us, so we could use the information in our continuing and broader responsibilities. The two-dimensional office practice had gained a third dimension.

We also wanted to identify exactly what was involved in developing "full-scope" primary care. First, there were more science, and new intellectual and analytical, skills, as well as a deeper understanding of disease and illness. The new practice was more of everything—more accountability, more knowledge, more sophisticated ways to address undifferentiated or complex illness, more understanding. Those who had attained this new level of practice knew that it was different but that the thousands of our MS-educated colleagues might not view the differentiation positively. For decades, our profession had been advocating nurse practitioners as a quality alternative to physicians in primary care. Policy and regulation had increasingly favored this plea by providing legal access and direct reimbursement to nurse practioners (NPs) for primary care, even though both continued to be limited. Partly because of the public's long-held view that physicians oversee or direct nursing care (and for most the nation's nurses this is true), and partly because nurses in practice did not have a doctorate, the hierarchy remained. Now we had a distinction among nurses that merited a doctoral degree title, and while this could help the new elites, it might come at the expense of the many without the new practice attributes and title. In many ways we believe that MS-prepared nurse practitioners are qualified to provide primary care. Nurses are remarkably able to sense nuanced signs of disease or a worsening condition, even when they may not have the full capability to name it or treat it. In this context, patients are not ill-served by selecting an NP for primary care; NPs may refer more, or—because they are better at it— they may care for more patients with chronic illness. But patients aren't at risk with an NP. The difference with the new practitioners is that they know more and can do more, and they can care for patients across sites of care. Both clinicians are fully qualified in the role their degree prepares them for. This isn't a case of an "A" team or a "B" team, but rather a situation where there is now a broader scope of practice and accountability for the nurse with the higher level of education.

Higher responsibility linked to higher education has always been true in the health professions. In the midst of this transition in nursing, we have a deep responsibility to articulate the continued value of traditional NPs. In the future, it is almost certain that the MS degree will not be an endpoint and that all nurses aspiring to graduate-level independent care roles will earn the clinical doctorate. It is this interim now, where we must be clear that competence in a given site, with clear responsibilities, can be provided by an NP with reliable high quality.

We were not only being challenged within our profession about the distinction between NPs and those with the clinical doctorate, but also by the charge that the clinical Doctor of Nursing Practice (DNP) was preparing mini-doctors. Although the majority of new clinical training comes from medicine, this was no different from the medical training that distinguished an NP from a bachelor's prepared nurse. Any new skills are adopted within a context of existing practice, and our context was nursing. The core elements of nursing and a nursing approach to care were not obliterated by gaining more knowledge of illness and disease, or the attendant sciences, which supported the new practice.

Coming closer to the overlap between generalist medicine and advanced clinical nursing—our vision of the DNP—gives nursing more credibility when taking on primary care as our domain. The more we knew that mirrored what primary care physicians knew, the better the argument to supplant them in this specialty. This was happening anyway by the gap left as physicians fled primary care careers, but we had a better chance of equal pay and equal authority for comparable practice if we could show we were, in fact, comparable.

While we contemplated and designed ways to paint a clear picture of this new clinical practice, our professional world was afire with new ideas that would compete with our vision. The University of Kentucky was already formulating a new degree in administration and systems management, which they called a Doctor of Nursing Practice. Other nursing schools, faced with stuffing new important training into already long and rigorous MS programs, (some with as many as 90 credits or 3 years of full-time graduate study) were contemplating some kind of new doctoral degree instead. A cascade of new medical knowledge fostered new specialties and subspecialties, and drew physicians into these practices, and away from generalist careers. There was an awakening everywhere that there were new frontiers in health care to grasp and secure, and nursing was responding. The Institute of Medicine (IOM), a policy organization for physicians and other health professionals, is one of the prestigious organizations within the National Academy of Sciences. In the late 1990s, the IOM embarked on a multiyear study to develop recommendations to increase the quality of medical care.

The first IOM report, issued in 1999, *To Err Is Human,* called for standards of practice to be redefined for the new century, and encouraged educational institutions to develop programs to meet these new and stronger standards. In 2001, the second report was published: *Bridging the Quality Chasm.* This report was far more specific about the standards required in the pursuit of quality. It recommended restructuring clinical education for physicians and for nurses, changing credentialing processes to reflect the current and emerging scope of care, and, importantly, distinguished the separate but important goals of clinical training and nonclinical administration and management.

That same year, several members of our nascent physician–nurse group developing the new degree for nurses presented a full-day workshop at the IOM on "Primary Care Quality." Our new role, and yet to be named degree, was the centerpiece of the "solutions" we presented in the workshop. Not surprisingly, most of the physicians in the audience didn't understand the nuanced but significant differences in this "new" nurse; the competencies of the new professional were difficult to portray. We found the clearest way was to describe case studies. Once the detail of a clinical encounter was made clear, some began to see how this new model with the cross-site accountability and deeper clinical knowledge was different. But with understanding, the old professional barriers rose immediately; this might be an improvement for nurses, but they still weren't doctors, nor could they substitute for them. This argument began to change from nurses can't be primary care doctors to a different question. The next year when I presented our model at a medical school seminar at the University of Wisconsin, one medical student in the audience asked, "Why should anyone go to medical school if they want to practice primary care?"

In 2005, the third IOM report was published: *The Bridge to Quality.* As an extension of the first two, this document set out a number of primary care competencies that would be linked to evidence-based care for certification. The reports made a clear call to change practice regulations so that all professionals would be able to practice at the highest level of their education and to rely on certification to assure competence.

While the IOM mission in these three reports was to fundamentally change health professions education and credentialing, nothing of importance has come from it. Certainly, there is more focus on evidence-based practice, and payers are well on the way to requiring evidence that a given intervention works before paying for it, but we are far away from the revolution the IOM report committees were anticipating. Nonetheless, it strengthened our case for the new degree in nursing, and we incorporated the competencies and curricula from the reports in our planning.

Recognizing that Columbia alone could not bring about national change, and understanding fully that our idea had to be replicable as well as admirable, we launched several initiatives to foster national adoption. We had been publishing articles and presenting our model at professional nursing meetings, as well as at several medical school and specialty society meeting. There was little backlash from specialists or even medical schools as the American Association of Medical Colleges (AAMC) published a positive article about the Columbia innovation in its journal for member medical schools. But nursing leadership across the country was skeptical and even hostile. Nursing schools had well-established MS programs in advanced practice, and to change could be financially and operationally difficult for them. And besides, they didn't have faculty know-how to make the transition. The only groups more inflamed than many in our own profession were the American Medical Association (AMA) and family practice physicians. For example, the New York State Medical Association president, Charles Aswad, had pledged openly to his membership that he would use all of his energies to shut down Columbia Advanced Practice Nurse Associates (CAPNA).

These physician groups actually need us if they intend to meet the nation's demand for primary care, but meeting that need doesn't seem to be their priority; sustaining barriers that protect MD-only authority in primary care appears to be more important to them. Perhaps they were worried that reimbursement would decrease for them and that in the future they might be paid at NP rates. But CAPNA was paid on the same fee schedule as physicians, and we planned to work toward pay equity for these new nurse clinicians wherever they practiced. It wasn't the fear of competition, or even the threat of lower payment, that fueled the AMA attacks. It was all about status. The idea that nurses could do what they did made their place in the medical hierarchy even lower than it already was.

The pushback from nursing was harder to manage. Their argument was essentially that the conventional master's degree NP was fully prepared to deliver primary care. They pointed to the hundreds of published articles attesting to NP competence and quality. We agreed with them. We were arguing for a new and higher level, something we initially called full-scope primary care, which was awkward and required lots of explaining. Deans were concerned their faculties weren't prepared to teach a new level of practice and that their influential alumni (most of whom would not return for an additional degree) might feel second class and make trouble or stop giving to the school. They worried that a longer educational program didn't guarantee any increase in salary or authority, so why would students even enroll? It was so much easier to simply say a new clinical degree was untenable and unnecessary.

But there was a palpable yearning for increased independence and recognition among nurses in practice, and particularly among the newest identifiable group of individuals contemplating a nursing career. This new nursing student either entered nursing as a college freshman, knowing about the clinical doctorate as a potential endpoint of his or her career, or is a mature second-career individual—someone who has already been trained for a different role in society and is now thinking about nursing. Both cohorts want an education where they can attain the same status and equity as other students who engage in graduate study for 4 or more years. If someone can become an MD in 4 years after college, why not a doctorate in nursing program for the same effort?

The University of Kentucky was insightful to see a market for nurses who wanted a doctoral degree, so they could be "doctor" among all the other "doctors" they worked with in their health care setting. And these nurses would be most attracted to a doctoral degree tied intimately to their profession, a Doctor of Nursing Practice, not a Doctor of Nursing Administration. Few nurses, however, enter their professional education aspiring to be administrators or systems administrators. They want to care for patients. In time, however, many reach a ceiling of authority and upward mobility unless they turn to administration. It is a sad commentary that many of our best and brightest clinicians have defaulted to nonpractice careers because of the lack of clinical advancement opportunities. The clinical doctorate could change that trajectory for these already in nursing and could provide the magnet to attract more new recruits to nursing. Over time, the nonclinical DNP may wither, as advanced clinical training may be more useful in moving up the hierarchy (even in nursing administration) than systems management training. But in 2000, there were enormous barriers to move the clinical doctorate ahead of new nonclinical DNP programs.

There was one group developed as a Columbia initiative that made all the difference, and this was the Council for the Advancement of Primary Care (CAPC). Using "access and quality" as our motto, Columbia invited 20 nursing and health policy leaders to join the council and work together to ensure that quality and standards would be developed for the new clinical doctorate. These members of CAPC (in the following list) have been instrumental in the presence and advancement of the clinical doctorate through all the tumult of the first 10 years of the new century, the decade when nursing experienced the colliding visions of the DNP degree.

CAPC MEMBERS

Kathleen Adreoli, DNS, Dean
Rush University College of Nursing

Geraldine Bednash, PhD, Executive Director
AACN

Robert H. Brook, MD, ScD Vice President
RAND Health

Richard A. Cooper, MD, Director
Health Policy Institute
Medical College of Wisconsin

Melanie Dreher, PhD, Dean
University of Iowa College of Nursing

Catherine Gilliss, DNSc, Dean
Yale University School of Nursing

Donna Hathaway, PhD, Dean
University of Tennessee at Memphis College of Nursing

Ada Sue Hinshaw, PhD, Dean
University of Michigan School of Nursing

Judy Honig, EdD, DNP, Associate Dean
Columbia University of School of Nursing

Robert Kane, MD, Professor
University of Minnesota School of Public Heath

Thomas Kean, Chair
9/11 Commission and
Former Governor of New Jersey

Kenneth Kizer, MD, President and CEO
National Quality Forum

Lucy Marion, PhD, Former President
NONPF

Mary O. Mundinger, DrPH, Dean
Columbia University School of Nursing

Lois Quam, CEO
Ovations, UnitedHealthcare

Marla Salmon, ScD, Dean
Emory University N.H. Woodruff School of Nursing

Joan Shaver, PhD, Dean
University of Illinois at Chicago College of Nursing

Patricia Starck, DSN, Dean
University of Texas at Houston School of Nursing

Reed Tuckson, MD, Senior Vice President
UnitedHealth Group

Myron Weisfeldt, MD, Chair, Medicine
Johns Hopkins University School of Medicine

Michael Whitcomb, MD, Senior Vice President
AAMC

Nancy Woods, PhD, Dean
University of Washington School of Nursing

The council met 15 times during that decade. Three of the meetings were held in New York City, but attendance was low at those meetings. The council members are all professionals with busy schedules and multiple responsibilities, and we therefore learned that an international location with interesting destinations where the members would want to visit drew the most attendees. There were two other reasons this worked well. Travel to a foreign country usually takes a stronger planning commitment than a trip to New York City, and being away in a different time zone discouraged the multitaskers on their cell phones from trying to stay connected while attending to council business. Members came, contributed fully, and became a remarkably collegial and supportive group of individuals, even when professional perspectives differed.

In our first meeting, held in Paris in June 2000, Columbia presentations stressed the cross-site and expanded accountability of the new level of nursing practice. Discussion focused on the overwhelming need for primary care and how this new nurse could meet that challenge. The American Association of Colleges of Nursing (AACN) and the National Organization of Nurse

Practitioner Faculty (NONPF) members recommended that the council consider uniform accreditation for this newly proposed degree that would "protect the public and unburden programs, faculty, and students from the multiple documentation and approval processes." Looking back, it is interesting to see how a distinctive certification was in our earliest discussions. We also discussed the new degree as a way to inspire a whole new generation of individuals to become nurses. We met again in New York City in January 2001 and spent time distinguishing the new doctorate from research doctorates. We were working toward a doctorate that would be distinguished as a higher level, independent, cross-site and standardized degree, one that would match a PhD researcher in substance as well as standing and would bring practice to the same level of training as research.

In January, NONPF announced it was forming a practice doctorate task force. A year later, in Phoenix in January 2002, the council held its third meeting. We further discussed the standards and scope we envisioned for the new degree. Nursing deans in the group had begun discussing plans for the new degree with their faculties (as had other nursing deans across the country), and following this meeting, Bednash decided that the AACN should also form a task force on the clinical doctorate.

In the fall of 2002, CAPC met in London. Two major concerns came out of the discussion. Most troubling was the major proliferation of doctoral degree planning focusing on administration, or leadership or systems management, not advanced clinical care. And, as the council continued to focus on standards and even certification, concern was raised as to whether we were assuming responsibilities that our professional organizations already held. Bednash noted that without AACN involvement the council's work in these areas would be "fringe." She noted that certification and accreditation organizations already existed and could accommodate the new degree without CAPC's efforts.

We knew AACN's involvement was critical and Bednash's participation had been (and would continue to be) invaluable. But we couldn't wait for existing organizations to survey the new programs and build a representative set of standards; we wanted *our* standards to set the pace. We believed the long and carefully evaluated model at Columbia—still being refined and evaluated—*was* the new standard. We didn't want it watered down by the conventional process of finding a common denominator among the deluge of new and variable programs. At the London meeting in 2002 we decided the best way to build standards was to define the essential competencies the new graduates should attain. Since competencies are the basis of curricula, we could see a plan evolving toward our goal if we could take this pathway.

The non-nurse members of the council began to challenge the deans: Quam noted that, "Nursing is a woman's profession that needs to redefine itself as something other than helping. You can lead the profession or be deans of nursing—stop trying to do both." She went on to say, "Using the same title for different competencies debases the currency. Medical care organizations won't spend the money to distinguish between these programs. Confusion is costly." Bednash warned that innovations can be seen as elitist, and that AACN could be a vehicle of acceptance for our ideas. Kizer called upon us to devote our efforts toward a better future system, as the recent IOM report (*Crossing the Quality Chasm*) set out, and not to force too much on the current environment. Cooper added, "Don't re-invent the Model T as family practice did." Furthermore, Cooper warned that "primary care has holes in it; get a new name."

Clearly, the discussion was recognizing the challenge of nonclinical doctorates that were being developed (University of Kentucky most prominently) which were in competition with (and causing potential confusion with) our proposed clinical doctorate. The council met again in New York City in December 2002. We circulated a vision statement for the council that promulgated the clinical doctorate degree incorporating competencies and standards. None of the other nursing deans would sign, deferring to the process still ongoing at Columbia where we were attempting to receive university approval for the degree, and none of the non-nursing members felt qualified—without nursing concurrence—to support a nursing degree. We were ahead of our friends once again. AACN reported that they were working on a draft on the practice doctorate for their January 2003 annual doctoral conference. Betty Lenz (a Columbia research faculty member who chaired the AACN committee) reported that the AACN draft document would focus on "commonalities of the clinical doctorate which includes advanced clinical practice." We were encouraged; if the AACN committee was equating "practice" with "clinical" perhaps they were arriving at the conclusion that would favor our brand of the DNP. After all, the AACN had formed a "practice" doctorate committee, and their draft referred to "clinical." In 2002 we had not yet decided what the title of the proposed degree would be at Columbia, but there were lots of discussions. We continued to more fully describe and promulgate the essential domains and competencies of a clinical DNP graduate. We began publishing doctoral competencies internally at Columbia, with circulation to leading nursing schools and organizations. The first formal set was completed in 2002 by Columbia clinicians who were practicing at this advanced level. This eight-page document included all of the domains and competencies already established by the NONPF, for MS programs, with additional competencies added that differentiate the DNP graduate. This document is titled "Full Scope Primary Care." The new doctoral competencies described the cross-site scope of care and more direct authority for all care. The ability to give care and exert decision making across sites of care was a fairly straightforward difference:

"… directs care in ambulatory, acute care, nursing homes …"

The remaining competencies differ from MS competencies in the stronger and more comprehensive wording used:

"Builds and maintains a therapeutic team ..."

"Diagnoses and manages acute and complex, co-morbid and chronic conditions"

"Rapidly assesses the patient's unstable and complex health care problems ..."

"Leads the interdisciplinary team ..."

"Orders, may perform, and interprets relevant complex diagnostic tests ..."

In order to show the difference and congruence with researchers, new areas of competency were described:

"Generates evidence from practice and applies data-mining techniques"

"Compares benchmarking statistics to practice standards to rate effectiveness of care"

Several of the new competencies described systems management, epidemiological skills, and sophisticated use of informatics. The document was a clear representation of clinicians who were passionately aware of their advanced practice and were trying to be specific where these advancements were distinguishable from MS-level education. Pushback from several NP groups was that they, too, practiced at this level, without a DNP degree. They believed that the basics of MS education had given them the tools to learn through experience after they earned their MS and joined the workforce.

We wanted more than the informal and spotty accomplishments that opportunistic practice opportunities offered. We wanted standards, a formal education to assure students learned the advanced skills, and the assurance that all of the components became essentials in the new level of practice: we wanted the educational formality and certification of these essentials that would capture the public's broad recognition and acceptance.

In August of 2003 the council met in Rome, in the hottest and most humid days of the year. Recognizing that the new practice we were promulgating was broader and deeper than conventional primary care, the council was renamed the Council for the Advancement of Comprehensive Care (CACC).

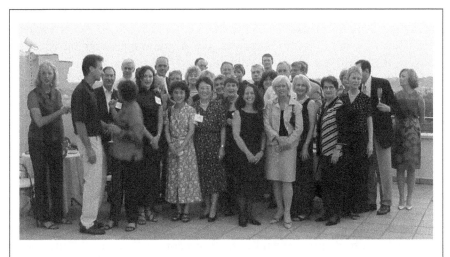

CACC Rome, Italy (2003)

●●●●●

The AACN document on the practice doctorate was circulated. They had come squarely in support of dual definitions of practice:

"Practice refers to direct care of patients *and* activities in support of direct care."

The draft goes on to state that specialized knowledge and skills needed for providers of direct care are quite different from skill set needed to determine strategies and systems. Is "direct practice" the same thing as "clinical practice?" Or, as some documents stated, does practice include all professional activities of nurses? Are they all "direct?" The meaning of "practice" was still evolving to stretch the canvas over the broadest set of nonresearch activities. We could see where the path was leading, but even if we adopted Doctor of Clinical Nursing as the title, for example, the distinction would not solve the problem if DCN and DNP were both "practice" doctorates. We certainly weren't going to say that our clinical encounters were not practice. The outcome was messy and unavoidable once practice was redefined.

In the efforts to be professionally inclusive—one of nursing's most tragic attributes—the professionally powerful, authentic, and core attributes of our profession were being redefined and eroded. Why would nurses want to confuse what practice is? It was difficult enough to titrate all the many levels of clinical care by nurses by different education levels. Now we were taking one new education level and confusing what the essential core of that degree would be, and in doing so, disassembling the meaning of one crucial word—practice—that we had agreed on since the profession first was established. None of nursing's competitors could have been clever enough to do what we were doing to ourselves. We at Columbia weren't giving up. We were so certain our idea was valuable, and that we would find a way to distinguish it.

Clearly, AACN could have done nothing other than to accept and promulgate the new definition of practice. Once programs across the country were developing programs in "practice" that focused on administration or leadership or other nonclinical outcomes, AACN had no choice but to include their programs as well as ours. Variability had been institutionalized.

Lucy Marion from NONPF also presented its draft on the "practice/professional/clinical doctorate," which would include "direct practice and health care leadership." They were following the same broad definitions of practice. In the month before the Rome meeting, NONPF and AACN held a doctoral forum to present and seek comment on their draft statements, which included the following comment:

the graduate of the practice doctorate will have in-depth clinical expertise, ability to link policy making with clinical systems, translate research into practice. ...

There were no descriptions of "in-depth clinical expertise" or what level of clinical training was required in a practice doctorate. There were lots of assumptions but not a lot of detail. Part of the discussion centered on whether advanced practice nurses could be grandfathered into the new title, suggesting that no new clinical education was required in a DNP other than MS-level training.

The document also included the statements: "Expected competencies for the various roles would need to be differentiated after the roles are defined," and "we endorse ... programs to include either or both direct and indirect practice while adhering to a consistent set of standards ... of core content ... supplemented by competencies specific to the domains of practice and specific roles." Direct practice would apparently be patient care, and indirect practice would be activities in support of patient care. This was the next step in parsing "practice" so that everyone could fit it and so as to preserve the idea that practice really was about patient care, and that one way or another, a nurse was "practicing" if engaged in any activity supporting the actual clinical delivery of care. Inclusivity, a self-defeating and restrictive hallmark of our profession, had been preserved. The other part of this tortured thinking is the idea that in designing the DNP degree, different roles should be determined first, and then they would all be clumped together into one degree, with distinction and recognition determined by roles rather than by the degree title. One person in the audience (no, not from Columbia) noted that the DNP degree could be "potentially disruptive if the proliferation of practice doctorates do not standardize title, curricula, and terminal competencies." The Nursing Doctorate (ND) degree had died from the lack of standards or terminal competencies, and those at the forum (AACN and NONPF as well as many attendees) were cognizant of that vulnerability with the DNP. However, the sense was that broad common standards would ensure that all DNP programs would be similar and that different competencies based on different roles would be minor issues. This idea teeters on a very unstable fulcrum; if the "standards" are broad enough, with very little specificity, the common product will be weak. The programs with the most to lose would be the clinical ones, since specificity about competencies matters most when the graduate is entrusted with the complex care of sick individuals. Broad standards that may or may not include sophisticated clinical acumen won't be sufficient to give the graduates firm standing to gain advanced authority and recognition in the clinical world.

The proposed commonalities in the degree would be systems, use of evidence, ethics, quality, and policy. These are what Judy Honig called "background" elements. She and her Columbia colleagues believed that the new clinical competencies were the "foreground" of a DNP degree. Others, however, saw it differently and believed that all DNPs would have the same in-depth sophisticated infrastructure, in addition to different "role" competencies in clinical care, or systems management or leadership.

The AACN statement continued: "We recognize that all programs offering the degree will produce graduates with somewhat different competencies." Apparently, this observation was no cause for concern.

At Columbia, we continued establishing a degree, which, in its focus on clinical sophistication, required the "background" elements that formed the "foreground" in nonclinical degrees. We knew that the clinical competencies exceeded those taught in MS programs, and we asserted they were at a level to merit a doctoral degree. We believed that a capstone project, equal to but different from a PhD dissertation, would solidify the doctoral title (although medicine and dentistry justify their doctorates without any special project). We were designing a portfolio of case studies, which evidenced the higher-level competencies as our capstone project. Capstone projects in nonclinical DNP programs were also being designed, but they were without standards; each school determines what a capstone project should entail.

With this one degree/variable competencies idea, we worried that the common denominator for the DNP would be far less, clinically, than if we had standardized one degree/standard competencies. And that lower common denominator would hurt our advancement in the clinical world. We believed this would pose barriers to establishing national standards for advanced clinical care and could result in less recognition and less authority. We continued to plead with an audience that was less and less interested in our arguments as the majority of the profession (and a majority of schools establishing the DNP) became comfortable with the variable new degree.

Other professions—medicine, law, dentistry, public health, business— all have essential distinguishing competencies required in their terminal degree (the highest degree in a discipline) programs. Why not nursing? It may be the perspective that nurses became nurses long before they became doctors, and therefore the doctoral degree can be granted without detailing any new nursing competencies; all that is needed is the addition of doctoral-level courses in support domains. This is what seems to be occurring with nonclinical DNP programs; nothing new in direct patient care knowledge or skill is necessary.

We understood why this decision was being made; we just didn't agree with it. During the Rome meeting, the CACC committee, which had worked on DNP competency standards since 2000, presented its work. Faculty from all CAPC nursing schools had participated: Rush University, University of Illinois at Chicago, University of Iowa, University of Texas at Houston, University of Washington, Yale University, and Columbia University.

New domains (accountability across sites of care, utilization and synthesis of evidence) were added as well as specific clinical skills. CACC discussed and confirmed the document, which described the differentiation of between MS and DNP competencies. Although CACC agreed on the differentiation between MS and DNP clinical competencies, this would not be part of the DNP degree requirements as it was playing out. Instead of repeating our arguments for common competencies in all DNP programs, we acknowledged the decisions being made within the profession. And so in January 2004 at a CACC meeting in New York City we formally adopted the DNP title in regard to the clinical doctoral work we were doing (including the Columbia decision to use the title) and now turned our attention to how else we could best distinguish and differentiate the clinical DNP graduates. During this same meeting CACC finally adopted a formal mission statement:

- Create a doctoral-level clinical role extending beyond traditional primary care
- Promulgate common core competencies
- Define a process to assure attainment of competencies (certification)
- Designate those who complete such certifications as Diplomates of the American Board of Comprehensive Care

Just as "practice" was getting redefined, we in the council were beginning to redefine primary care as comprehensive care. We continued to define and build competencies for what we were calling "full-scope" care.

As an important part of the follow-up to the meeting, we sent information about our work in progress and the council goals to several external organizations, including Kaiser Permanente, UnitedHealthcare, the U.S. Health and Human Services offices of Medicare and Medicaid, AARP, and several pharmaceutical companies.

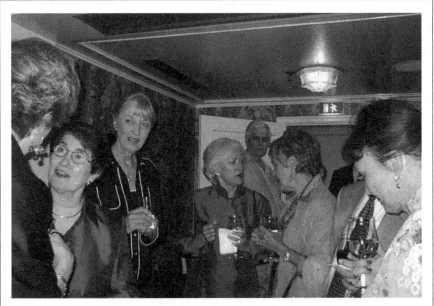

CACC cocktail party in Norway (2004).
Left to right: Ada Sue Hinshaw, Joan Shaver, Mary Mundinger, Bob Kane,
Polly Bednash, and Melanie Dreher

● ● ● ● ●

In June 2004, Columbia University approved the DNP degree, just days before the council's meeting in Bergen, Norway. Five of the deans of CACC nursing schools represented in the council reported that their faculties were establishing DNP degree programs. Only two—Columbia and the University of Tennessee at Memphis—developed a clinical DNP program. Tennessee, under the innovative and charismatic deanship of Michael Carter, had been moving toward this level of practice for several years. They had by necessity placed it under their DNSc degree program, while making every effort to distinguish their DNSc program from all others across the United States, which were research degrees. This was a deeply frustrating solution for Carter, who developed his own cross-site practice as an NP while he was dean. Faculty following his lead knew they were onto something different and more advanced than MS-level clinical skills as well as being distinct from a research degree. Carter would have chosen to give a new title—a new doctoral title—to the model he was designing, but he did not have that choice. The state of Tennessee would not allow a doctoral program and title to be registered and to grant degrees, unless such title was already established in another state; a curious and conservative policy. Carter was a leader constrained by a nonleadership environment. Nonetheless, he celebrated with us all, magnanimous and full of humor as always, but you could tell it rankled him. He had lived the beginning of this transition in his own school and in his own practice. While his idea was more informal than what unfolded at Columbia, he had been breaking new ground. The University of Tennessee now has a DNP program.

The other CACC schools developing DNP programs that were not focused on advanced clinical training had lots of company. Nearly all the new DNP programs were meeting the systems/management competency standards. I don't believe these deans' continued and highly participatory work on the council was at odds with the decisions they made in the schools they led. They believed in, and supported, a strong distinctive clinical DNP; they just didn't have clinical resources or faculty support to do so in their own schools.

Columbia had agreed to the AACN distinctions on practice because we did not want to be an outlier and because we believed—still believe—that clinical DNP programs will in time be the only DNP programs. Our profession continues to shorten the time it takes to earn a first degree in nursing (1 year for college graduates studying nursing for the first time), and now collapses MS and DNP education into a single degree—the DNP. In this same year (2004), the AACN membership voted that all advanced practice nursing would be at the doctoral level by 2015. This sounds like a breathtakingly short transition, but since most nurses believed a DNP degree was MS-level clinical plus supporting courses, one can understand that such a plan would not be that difficult to achieve. If all advanced practice education will occur only in doctoral programs in the future, the clinical DNP is much more likely to thrive. By taking away MS degree endpoints, the DNP clinical programs can become standardized; albeit at the conventional MS levels of practice only the title would change. A nonclinical DNP program, focused on management or systems, will either have no advanced clinical component or a doctoral-level clinical component. Therefore, if clinical training has to be taught at the doctoral level (MS-level programs will no longer be available), why not teach the clinical component in every program at the highest level possible? And if clinical training in all DNP programs is alike, why have two kinds of DNP programs?

Time is on our side for another reason. As more clinical DNPs graduate and practice in a variety of settings across the country, their practice will become more identifiable and more accessible; they will be practicing and teaching in programs where their expertise can guide students and faculties in achieving the new higher-level clinical competencies.

In addition, future recruits to nursing doctoral programs will be far more attracted to clinical practice or research than to the more oblique management endpoints. Those in management positions today (without a doctorate) want a degree that matches their current interests and one where they don't have to leave that position to revert to a clinical arena to earn the degree. Nonclinical DNP programs meet that need. But if all advanced practice programs are taught at the doctoral level in the future, then DNP graduates who aspire to management careers will have already achieved clinical training at the doctoral level. The only weakness in this design is if DNP clinical training for advanced practice is taught at different levels in different programs. The way things are now, some DNP programs recognize MS-level advanced practice as sufficient and add only the infrastructure courses in "indirect" practice. Other programs, like Columbia's, offer indistinguishable or very similar "indirect" practice courses, but also add a higher level of clinical training. The differences between these two kinds of DNP programs rest on differences in clinical competency. Although nursing has agreed that MS programs in advanced practice will end by 2015 and that all advanced practice will be taught at the doctoral level, there is still an unanswered question: Do all DNP programs have to teach advanced practice? If so, why shouldn't all DNP programs have the same high clinical component? It's only a matter of time we keep telling ourselves; if you're heading in the right direction, a Buddhist saying has it, just keep walking. Clinical care will only get more complex, more sophisticated. The systems and leadership expertise will always be needed, but the clinical core of the DNP will increasingly become sophisticated and standardized.

During the fall of 2004 and early 2005, faculty completed the DNP program, still pending university approval, and we celebrated the graduation of these premier clinicians. We even designed a new hood for DNP doctoral candidates—the peach for nursing was preserved but was bordered with an ever so subtle dark green braid. We were saying, "We are nursing doctors with a touch of medicine." It was mostly just a touch of fun in the midst of our landmark achievement.

In June 2005, the council met in Prague, one the most magnificent cities in Europe. We had an international presence as we had earlier in council meetings, with attendees from Australia, Canada, Sweden, and the UK. DNP education was already being discussed in academic centers in these countries. In the Prague meeting, we finally changed the content of the this new clinical practice from "full-scope" primary care to "comprehensive care," to match the name of the Council for the Advancement of Comprehensive Care—CACC. We thought some of the family practice physicians might call us "quacks" because of the sound of "CACC," but they never did.

As the council—and our new practice—became more established within a comprehensive format, we worked with AACN in their new recommendation for advanced practice specialty designations. Over the years, faculties in nursing had developed ever new and narrowly focused specialties, finally numbering near 100. As with the AACN decision to promulgate different role specialties in the DNP—essentially clinical or nonclinical (but supposedly in support of clinical care)—they also were attempting to redefine advanced practice into four broad categories of clinical focus, with subspecialty training part of role differentiation. We at Columbia were determined to make comprehensive care one of the four. We succeeded, and comprehensive care became the only advanced practice specialty that educates clinicians for cross-site care. The others are family, women and children, and adult. We therefore had a category for advanced practice that described the clinical DNP. But in the years to come there would be problems with maintaining this distinction. Although all existing advanced practice programs currently at the MS level are required to morph into the doctoral degree programs by 2015, there is no plan to upgrade the clinical level of DNP education to the comprehensive care competencies CACC was developing. Was it possible that as this transition occurred, there would be two levels of clinical DNP programs? A dual meaning (clinical and nonclinical) in the degree was already problematic; further differences within the clinical DNP programs could pose a huge barrier to public understanding and recognition of the graduates of the more sophisticated clinical DNP programs. With increased variability would come confusion and the chance that the more advanced clinical programs would never take root.

As CACC contemplated this potential, we turned our attention—as we had discussed at the very beginning of our discussions in 2000—to certification as the key distinguishing credential at Columbia. As part of this intensified effort to develop competencies as the standard for a clinical DNP graduate, we published a book in 2005 titled, *Case Studies: The Doctor of Nursing Practice Setting a New Standard in Health Care.* The Hope Heart Institute published and disseminated the book. Phil Nudelman, CEO of the institute, was also chairman of Columbia Nursing's Board of Visitors, and he oversaw the publication. With several newly minted DNP graduates as the authors, case studies, which had been part of their portfolio of 15, were published as chapters in the book. They are—still—stunning in their depth, complexity, and brilliance. By showcasing the best and most diverse of our faculty's work, we no doubt raised questions among our readers about how long and difficult it might be for a nursing faculty to develop a program that could develop similarly talented graduates. Perhaps we should have published case studies that met doctoral criteria but described cases a novice DNP graduate could expect to accomplish in practice. In our pride to show what seasoned NPs with a clinical doctorate could do, we missed a large part of our audience: faculty who wanted to develop a program like ours.

We asked a distinguished Columbia physician colleague to write the Foreword for the book. Joseph Tenenbaum, the Edgar M. Leifer Professor of Clinical Medicine, had been part of the cohort who taught and mentored our pioneer faculty class. He wrote, in part, about these new clinicians: "How do they stand apart from the work of young physicians completing the Doctor of Medicine? They emerge as integrating the science and current practice with a disciplined interest in the evidence that underscores it." He goes on to say, "In this era of greater specialization, the ease with which a patient with complex problems is shuttled into a singular diagnostic category because of the proclivity of the physician is too familiar. The Doctors of Nursing Practice shun such ready narrowness. Furthermore, the extraction of the individual from the disease is rarely seen in the reports; the Doctor of Nursing Practice is empowered to view the patient in the context of illness. Whether perspective will be altered as interaction in the medical model continues is unclear; generally, the firm foundations they have entered with will provide a buttress against reductionism."

The back cover of the book is filled with quotes from other nationally known nurses and physicians. Universally, their statements show an expectation that these new clinicians will enhance and change primary care. Now we had to fulfill those expectations by distinguishing them from the well-meaning and highly educated nurses with the same academic degree who would not have these skills.

16

· · · · ·

Back on the Home Front

· · · · ·

DURING THESE EARLY AND TUMULTUOUS years of degree development and distinction, Columbia nursing was thriving and changing. In 2000 the hospital closed our innovative Center for Advanced Practice (CAP). There was no lessening of demand for patient care at the practice, but the hospital's structure for clinics for the underserved had changed to return to the old model of rotating medical residents providing privacy care. Our CAP clinicians easily found other practices but missed their collegial and exciting independent setting. Interestingly, as our 4 years of faculty practice had demonstrated, there were far more opportunities to join specialty practice—and provide primary care to specialty patients—than to find a pure primary care setting. In 2000, all nurse practitioner faculty in practice, except for Columbia Advanced Practice Nurse Associates (CAPNA), were in specialty practices.

We continued to do well financially. Each year 20% of our revenues were unspent and were invested in our endowment, which was rapidly growing. In 2000, we reached $33 million. That year's budget was $14 million, with $5 million from the National Institutes of Health (NIH) grants. Our researchers were carrying the day for us. While practice monies subsidized full-time appointments, research actually made money for us. This same year we opened an Office of Research Resources in the school to provide support for grant writing, hiring grant supported staff, and generally giving an identity to our investigators.

The year 2001 was clouded for all of us by the 9/11 tragedy; it had happened in our city, with the clouds of smoke and destruction hanging over our enterprise directly up the Hudson River. We welcomed our new president that year and shared in the rededication those seminal events foretold.

In 2002, we reached—for the first time—the goal of all research faculty: each one achieving external funding support for their studies. The senior investigators continued to receive NIH or prestigious foundation awards, and several junior faculty began their promising path on the funding ladder with

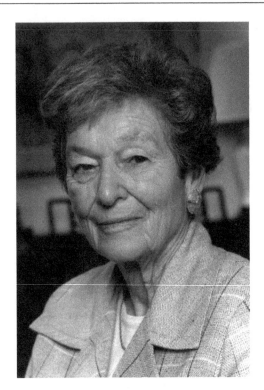

*Mary Dickey Lindsay (1995) alumna
of the century.*

• • • • •

competitive and prestigious grants from the provost's Strategic Research Fund. Each was burnishing nursing's standing within the university as well as with external organizations. This same year we announced the establishment of two new endowed chairs. One was the gift of Mary Dickey Lindsay, our most dedicated and distinguished alumna, honoring her lifelong commitment to women's health. The second chair was also in honor of an alumna, Dorothy Rogers, who had been an administrator early in the school's history. In 2002, we had a total of 22 faculty (two thirds of the full faculty) engaged in faculty practice. As the pattern was to continue, they were primarily in specialty departments in Columbia's medical school: radiology, organ transplant, neurology, pediatrics, anesthesia, and obstetrics. We had fewer Entry to Practice (ETP) enrollees as the nursing shortage continued to constrain our hospital training sites.

Our old and insufficient building continued to be an obstacle to our initiatives. We had received over $1.5 million in gifts toward the new building and had a rapidly growing unrestricted endowment to commit to a new building, but there was no institutional commitment for us to make firm plans to get in the queue for debt financing. Meanwhile, we watched our competitors build new, bigger buildings at Hopkins, Michigan, and Penn.

In 2003, we continued to seek ways to wrest approval from the university for a new building. We contracted with an architectural firm—Urbane Architects—to discuss building plans. They gave us estimates of $29 million to restore our existing building, or $45 million to build a new, bigger one on the same land. We projected using $25 million of our unrestricted endowment and borrowing the remaining $20 million from the university. Even at 7% for 25 years, the annual cost was less than half of our recurring surplus. Financially, this made a strong argument, but the university still would not allow us to use the university debt service. If we could have done so, we would have gone to a commercial lender who would have seen us as a good investment. But of course that was out of the question.

In 2003, our ETP enrollment doubled as we found new and more welcoming clinical training sites for students. Even with this huge increase in tuition revenues, our reliance on tuition went below 60% of all revenues for the first time in the school's history. Researchers continued to hit the ball out of the park, gifts and endowment income grew, and training grants for programs gave us new resources. By the end of the year, we had 30 faculty in practice and 16 research grants for 12 research faculty. We had made significant investments in technology for both faculty and students. Sue Bakken was awarded the first NIH grant the school had ever received, one that would support core resource development for research grants.

In 2004, with gifts, investment of unspent income, and a healthy growth of the university endowment, ours reached $40 million. Even with our strong financial position, we continued to protest our unfair common cost assessment. We were paying 19% of our revenues, whereas medicine paid only 9%, public health 11%, and dentistry 14%. The bigger the school budget, the less proportion of revenues went to common costs. There is some argument for this, but not enough to support our tax. We had more faculty in practice (using practice site resources, not the school's), and our space was tiny. Still, the tax was sustained.

The number of applicants to our ETP class was the largest since the program began; we had over 500 applicants for 50 spaces. And this was even more stunning since the 1-year cost of the program—$93,000—was so high. We projected a fund balance of unspent revenues at $8 million for the year—with expenditures at $20 million. It all went into the endowment.

The Doctor of Nursing Science (DNSc) program was in its tenth year. We had very few enrollees and even fewer graduates. The first three to finish the program did not pursue research careers, but took positions of clinical leadership that were not that different from what they had held before the degree. Our requirement for full-time study was not attractive to students. Our researchers were only recently being awarded grants that included stipends for doctoral students, and even then a student's annual income would be far less than what they earned in the positions they held when they applied to the program. Our idea was that the only way to think and act successfully as a researcher was to be immersed in that work as a student. We didn't think part-time study over 5 to 6 years would yield the same outcome. But we weren't attracting postbaccalaureate students, and as history had shown, nursing doctoral students had usually been in their professional careers for years before considering graduate study. They weren't interested in devoting themselves to a poorly financed full-time student role.

Even as we struggled with full-time DNSc study, we determined that our Doctor of Nursing Practice (DNP) program would only admit full-time students. We did so for the same reasons—success in the new role would require a dedicated educational involvement. Students who continued in their pre-DNP practices posed a serious learning barrier. We belived that learning a new role while practicing only the old one would hamper required assumption of the new skills, perspective, and responsibility. This time we would start with a faculty cohort positioned to mentor our students. Our about-to-be DNP faculty all had positions where they practiced in their new roles, and it would be easy to accommodate the small DNP class size in the clinical sites.

We began 2005 with excitement and high hopes. We graduated our first DNP class; all of them our faculty. The physicians who had mentored them all came to graduation, and when the new DNPs went to their practice sites that week flowers were on their desks, new white coats with their name and new title hung on their doors, and business cards were on their desks. The doctors were proud of their new doctors.

Our revenues continued to exceed our costs. In part this was the enormous success of our researchers, in part the subsidy of practice salaries, in part our booming enrollments. We were bursting at the seams in our little building, but we were saving a lot of money. That year we added $11.5 million of unspent income to our endowment. We also received approval to give raises, which were 8% above university guidelines. Our only concerns were the inadequate space we occupied and the growing gap between our DNP program and the cascade of nonclinical DNP programs appearing around the country. We wanted our new model to be mainstream. We knew it was more difficult and challenging to succeed with our DNP brand, but we believed it was the right challenge and worth the difficulty; we were changing nursing, we were filling the outlines of our profession with a robust and dazzling practice. We had to find ways to distinguish—and then grow—this innovation.

Section V

Certification and Competence: 2005–2010

སྙན་པོ་། སྒྲ་མདངས་སྒྲིག་པོ།

17
•••••

Certification and Residency: Establishing DNP Clinical Practice Competency
•••••

THIS LAST PERIOD IN MY deanship, though enriched by 20 years of seasoning and success, was the most contentious of all. This was true for two reasons. First, our practice advancements were becoming increasingly threatening to conventional generalist physicians and their organizations. Caring for Medicaid patients in a new and sophisticated way in a medical center environment had caused some grumbling and concern. But, after all, these patients were poor people with inadequate status and reimbursement, and Columbia was just carrying out a demonstration project. The arrival of Columbia Advanced Practice Nurse Associates (CAPNA) on the scene 3 years later caused serious consternation because these were mainstream patients with commercial reimbursement. But still this was just New York City and didn't affect those physicians who were outside this rarified metropolis. The resulting Doctor of Nursing Practice (DNP) clinical degree caused more conflict and uproar in nursing education than in the field of general medical practice. Conservative medical groups had no standing in this movement, and no clear understanding of how this would fundamentally impact their heavily protected distinction. I don't think organized medicine recognized that a clinical doctorate in nursing could so radically reduce the boundaries of their oversight of nursing. No longer was the scope of nursing viewed as a circle within the larger circle of medicine; now the two circles overlapped, and the common areas of that overlap were large and growing. Physicians never saw the power of the DNP nurses emerging, although they were not happy with nurses being called doctor.

In the period 2005–2010, however, the incremental assumption of nursing independence in primary care went national, and medicine's response went viral. This occurred as a result of the establishment of a national certification program for DNP graduates who had the new and sophisticated clinical skills. The angry and often vicious response from medicine was inflamed and fueled by the fact that the certification was offered by the same organization that certified MDs for a license to practice. It was more than they could bear.

The second area of contention that was brewing in this period was the continued, and increasingly unacceptable, delay by the university in approving our long-held plans for a new building. This had simmered since the day Maxwell Hall came down, before I became dean. But it had been a central part of my plan since the day I took office. Early on, there were more urgent issues, and then there was the fundamental need to show we had the stable finances to pay for a building, and the delays as the university struggled with its own financial downturn, unable and unwilling to approve debt financing, even to a triple A entity such as ours. Finally, I made the issue one of my primary goals, with the support of faculty, donors, and several influential trustees. But by then the president had essentially given approvals and oversight of the health sciences schools to the vice president of health sciences, and he was as determined to say no to my ultimatum as I was to make it. The outcome was foreordained. The school would not, on my watch, get a new building. It's still not clear why his approval was not forthcoming, but there are many possible reasons.

PLANS AND RATIONALE FOR DNP CERTIFICATION

The plans for certification, however, went forward. The National Organization of Nurse Practitioner Faculty (NONPF) published their practice doctorate final document in October 2006. NONPF apparently believed additional direct care clinical skills were not needed in DNP clinical programs where the students were already certified MS-level nurse practioners (NPs). They skipped over how NPs get the clinical skills they attribute to DNPs. Their document states: "A nursing practice doctoral program for nurse practitioners shall prepare the fully accountable independent health care provider with expert standing in the delivery and/ or management of evidence-based health care to patients *across health care settings*. The nurse practitioner with a practice doctorate will provide care to patients *with increasingly complex health care needs*" (italics added). Since these italicized competencies are not part of conventional NP curricula or outcomes, how do the DNP graduates achieve them? The statement never describes how these new competencies are attained and never states that such training should be included in DNP programs. The American Association of Colleges of Nursing (AACN) statements similarly glaze over the advanced clinical competencies of a DNP graduate, leaving that determination to existing NP credentialing organizations. No organization wanted to land on this crucial square in the new game of DNP: How do conventional MS programs in advanced practice become clinical DNP programs where graduates demonstrate a new level of clinical practice?

All of the organizations were confident in describing the systems management, evidence-based learning, ethical, and quality "essentials," but the practice essential was left for someone else (or everyone else) to decide for themselves. NONPF even warns against premature "random standards."

ARE CONVENTIONAL ADVANCE PRACTICE NURSING MS PROGRAMS CAPABLE OF PREPARING FULL-SCOPE PRACTICE GRADUATES AT THE DOCTORAL EXPERTISE LEVEL?

NONPF also published a document in 2006 titled "Practice Doctorate Nurse Practitioner Level Competencies." Twenty-three representatives of nursing schools or nurse credentialing agencies participated in the development of this document, which states in part that existing NP programs already have "core competencies" that produce NPs capable of "full scope of practice as a licensed independent practitioner." Did that mean NP programs teach "full-scope" cross-site authority for care? That was news to us. These skills and authority are not taught in NP programs, nor are these competencies tested in NP certification exams.

We were dismayed that our organizations wanted to consider conventional training of NPs as equivalent to our new and detailed doctoral-level practice. It was dangerous, however, to take on the proud thousands of NPs, or hundreds of nursing scholars, who wanted to believe there was nothing new to learn in clinical care. While nursing organizations were morphing standards to include cross-site care, more authority, and knowledge to care for complex patients, these standards did not include the necessary education to achieve these competencies. To us this appears to be lack of courage on the part of these organizations, not lack of knowledge. They were acknowledging higher standards and ignoring what it takes to get there. And of far greater importance than the marginalization of the Columbia model, it placed serious constraints on developing justifiable high standards for the new practice doctorate and for the graduates.

Interestingly, Bednash and AACN have continued to work with us and with the Council for the Advancement of Comprehensive Care (CACC). They don't deny that the clinical expertise in the Columbia program exceeds what is being taught in MS education, but they advocated a DNP model whereby our distinctive practice was only one of the many ways to "practice." Bednash is too savvy to join the forces that were saying NPs already had the clinical acumen of DNPs. She, too, supported standards for DNP education; she just parsed practice in a way that we found to be alien, leaving those distinctions to be met within the variable DNP degree outcomes. Her honesty, however, and her standing, were instrumental in CACC's cohesiveness and our campaign to establish a national certification for our brand of doctoral practice.

MOVING TOWARD A PRACTICE CERTIFICATION EXAM
WITH THE NATIONAL BOARD OF MEDICAL EXAMINERS

CACC met in St. Petersburg, Russia, in the spring of 2006 where we first discussed the potential of working with the National Board of Medical Examiners (NBME) to develop a certification exam. We could see that because of the variability of the DNP programs (20 were already established), the most promising, and quickest, way to distinguish clinical DNP graduates was to do so through certification. Even before nonclinical DNP programs evolved, as early as the 2002 London CACC meeting, physician members Mike Whitcomb, Buz Cooper, and Ken Kizer were all urging us to focus on competencies, not the degree. That may be because everyone in medicine has the same degree, and distinction in the various medical specialties is earned by distinguishing competencies through certification. Regardless of why they gave this advice so early in the development of this advanced clinical, they were right.

We had several options in developing a certification exam:

- We could leverage existing MS specialty certifying exams to add new competencies to be tested for DNP candidates, but that would have been a lifetime project. First, we would have had to convince them, and their constituencies, that there actually was a new higher level of competence than the scope of an MS prepared nurse. We had little chance of winning that argument. The embedded and conservative belief that DNP clinical was nothing new would continue as accepted wisdom, and it would take years (maybe decades) before existing certification exam organizations recognized a change in practice, reflected in the more comprehensive DNP clinical practice, and then—only then—change their exams to incorporate this new learning and practice. There were over 100 certifying groups for advanced practice in nursing, and convincing them all would take years.
- A second option was to build the new exam with a more generic certification organization. This would have required us to develop all the questions for this exam. That we could have done since we had competency-specific questions in all of our DNP courses at Columbia. But it takes years— maybe 10—and several hundred test takers to validate a new exam. We simply didn't have that much time or resources to carry out such a long investment period. Nor would we have the large numbers of test takers needed for test validation for several more years.
- The third option was to partner with an existing credentialing organization, which already had a pool of validated questions that covered the new DNP competencies. That led us straight as an arrow to NBME. Not that we didn't have several concerns: Should we ally the DNP certification directly with a medical organization? Were we leaving nursing? Would nursing organizations and schools be distanced from us and consider us an outlier? And, importantly, would NBME work with us?

Don Melnick, president of NBME, proved to be the fourth distinguished physician hero during these 25 years who had the courage—and who shared our vision—to support our radical ideas. Melnick was not only willing to work with us to develop a DNP exam, but he was an active, insightful, and spirited partner. He knew there would be serious and sustained disagreement and lobbying from physician organizations, but like Weisfeldt before him, he simply told his constituents it was the right thing to do, that physicians should welcome the high standards DNPs would have to meet in passing the exam, standards that would benefit patients and medicine. He also reminded his medical constituents that NBME already was in the business of developing certifying exams for professions other than medicine, and that their mission was to continue developing the highest and most reliable standards for practitioners of all health professions who sought their assistance in developing competency exams.

Melnick also wisely counseled us on how we could develop an exam that might come from a pool of some questions and might test comparable practice without being an equivalent exam. Equivalent became the "E word" which we danced around carefully, while nonetheless crafting an exam

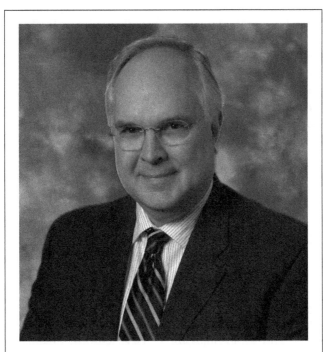

Dr. Don Melnick, president of the National Board of Medical Examiners.

• • • • •

that would test the same competencies as a newly minted MD would have attained. This "sameness" was crucial to understanding the function of nurses and primary care. Since 1986 at Columbia, and long before that in my own mind and writing, it was clear that to equally participate in care, with comparable authority and pay, nurses must without question, show their care was comparable.

How better to do that than to essentially take the same qualifying exam? One would not be required to earn the DNP degree (the medical exam is required for the MD degree), but would be required for the as-yet-to-be-standardized authority and recognition for these new comprehensive care providers.

We did not want to limit DNP clinical certification to just the exam derived from the NBME pool for the MD licensing exam. We wanted to establish a multifaceted set of requirements that would include more than an exam and that would recognize the competency achievements in nursing that precede DNP education.

INTRODUCTION OF THE DNP CLINICAL RESIDENCY

At the St. Petersburg meeting, we presented our plan to the CACC membership for a DNP exam to be developed by NBME, and we concurrently presented a plan for a clinical residency for DNP students, which included the development of a portfolio attesting to the attainment of the new competencies. Therefore, in our plan, DNP certification would require MS certification as an advanced practice nurse, plus a DNP degree, plus a residency (perhaps within the DNP degree, or perhaps post-DNP) and finally, the exam. In this decision we did two things. We acknowledged MS-level competency as essential in the full skill set of a DNP, and we defined the differences between the two. We took this step because it recognized our base in conventional advanced practice nursing and also helped explain why we chose NBME to develop an exam to test the added competencies, nearly all of which came from medicine.

The addition of the residency and its components was an attempt to merge the new medically oriented competencies with those that were more nursing specific. We did this in order to arrive at a certification that not only recognized the new medical skills, but also combined those skills to forge a new nursing practice that was distinctive from, and in many ways additive to, general practice in medicine.

During the entire development of DNP clinical practice we debated what to call the scope of practice achieved by the graduates. Primary care already had meaning, even though it was somewhat blurred. In most people's minds, primary care was outpatient office encounters with a clinician who could resolve less serious conditions, or refer the more acute or urgent ones to a specialist. Primary care was the first contact most patients would make in the health care system for ongoing health maintenance, prevention, and care for symptomatic illness. MDs and NPs have been practicing this brand of primary care for decades. DNPs could do more, and we labeled this comprehensive care. They could provide care to more complexly ill patients, in the hospital and ER as well as in the office, and most importantly, they could provide seamless care, advice, and coordination along this continuum. DNP education was also an extension in knowledge and care in other specialties where nurses had already achieved MS-level certification, such as acute care, or midwifery, or anesthesia. Even with this broad scope of comprehensive skills and knowledge, we kept our focus on advancing DNPs in the narrower one of "primary care." This is where the battle would be fought for nursing recognition and authority. This is where the profound and visible shortage lies. The public, the government, specialist physicians, and the payers all want to solve the primary care deficit. If DNPs can show their reliable comparability there, it will open doors for all DNPs in the future. So we continued to focus on DNP competence in primary care—we could do what physicians do in that specialty—while we were, in fact, developing a far broader and deeper role for nurses in health care. Comprehensive care as evidenced by clinical DNPs, is not only advanced clinical care across sites of care; it is also a model that incorporates cost-effective strategies, individualized care that utilizes evidence-based approaches, and added knowledge of business, legal, and ethical parameters of care. In time, our new "brand" would be the preferred one. Without losing sight of this goal, we continued to clarify for the public that DNPs are the primary care clinicians of the future.

In our certification plan, we envisioned the residency as a devoted clinical year of sophisticated practice caring for a panel of patients in all sites where they received care. It would consume about half the time and credits for a post-MS degree. If DNP graduates in a nonclinical program wanted to then attain the higher level clinical role, they could participate in a residency post-DNP. We envisioned the residency as required in a clinical DNP program or as a voluntary postdoctorate experience for nonclinical DNP graduates. We viewed the portfolio as a set of sophisticated case studies that would attest to competency development and prepare the graduate for an exam that would test that knowledge. The exam was the third and final requirement for certification. This tripartite set of requirements was presented to CACC: MS certification as an advanced practice nurse, DNP degree with residency, and exam. The council members—especially the nurse members—liked the connection and requirement of MS advanced practice as an integral part of DNP certification. Everyone on the council (with some reservations by the nurse members) was in favor of an exam developed by NBME. They agreed that the organization was held in high regard, and we would benefit from their reputation and standards. There was some concern among the nurse members regarding not only the use of a medically oriented exam, but also our not seriously considering contracting with nursing certification organizations that also had high standards and reliable exams. We agreed with this assessment except for one large gap: Nursing organizations had not developed or standardized reliable questions to cover this new level of practice. NBME already had that pool of exam questions.

CACC FAILS TO APPROVE THE DNP RESIDENCY REQUIREMENT

The council agreed with our plan except for the residency. The sense was that our residency had meaning for programs aiming at the certification we described, but that so few programs were moving in that direction and it was too prescriptive. They did continue to believe that the sophisticated cross-site practice we had developed was different from conventional MS-level practice, but that all DNP graduates should be eligible for the proposed certification as long as they were also advanced practice nurses. Because of the lack of common experiences and standards for DNP programs, and the high level of competence some NPs had developed after their master's degree, it was possible for graduates to meet the new competency standards and pass the proposed exam without a specific and narrowly defined residency. The council decision was that a residency would not be required for certification, but that further development of residency content and achievements would be valuable. Several members noted that the residency could become a useful and voluntary experience for DNP graduates as preparation for the certification exam if their DNP program had not included this advanced clinical training.

CACC was established as an advisory group, and we needed to establish a separate and independent group to actually offer the certification. During the 2006 meeting we began to discuss such a board, and we approved working with NBME to develop an exam.

COMPETENCIES OF A CLINICAL NURSING DOCTORATE (THIRD EDITION)

In 2006, Columbia nursing published the third edition of "Competencies of a Clinical Nursing Doctorate." It was presented and discussed at CACC and, as in the first two editions, competencies new to doctoral practice were distinguished within the overall role of comprehensive care. The new practice emerges even more sharply in this document, which states that DNPs

"develop, direct, and deliver comprehensive care to patients with acute, chronic, and complex illness"

"determine the need for inpatient admissions or emergency evaluation and actively manage, co-manage, and coordinate care"

"develop and implement diagnostic strategies and therapeutic interventions across settings..."

"formulate diagnostic strategies to deal with ambiguous or incomplete data in developing differential diagnoses"

Determining evidence-based outcomes of care and employing cultural, epidemiologic, and genetic determinants of health and disease were all listed as specific competencies in the new level of practice.

A few months later, CACC and Columbia hosted an invitational conference in New York City on how to set up a clinical DNP program. All CACC schools and several others came, presented their views, and discussed ways in which this new degree could best be supported. Not surprisingly, there was a broad belief that all DNP programs would advance clinical care without requiring the defined sophisticated clinical education that Columbia was advocating. No one was against our model; there just weren't a lot of aspirants to do what we were doing, nor did they think it was necessary. Certifications are a good thing, they agreed, but nursing organizations would evolve their certification exams incrementally as new knowledge or scope of practice became apparent and became the norm. There was wide acknowledgment that the profession had reached doctoral-level accomplishments that were different from those achieved by researchers. This new level—the new doctoral level—could be earned by applying existing clinical care knowledge with the addition of advanced system management, new technologies, and new and refined administrative strategies. There was no sense of urgency to establish a new certification program.

Most believed that the education in MS advanced practice had grown in scope and sophistication over the years, and now merited a doctorate, as long as the new management skills were added. There was great reluctance to accept the Columbia model as the clinical competency standard beyond what NPs were acquiring in conventional NP programs.

Many in the profession worked hard to convince themselves (and others) that a DNP degree did not necessarily require standards for a new level of clinical knowledge or scope of care. That graduates of the new degree would achieve variable competencies in their degree programs was not a concern. The fact that "practice" in nursing now had a blurred meaning, with inclusiveness blotting out distinctiveness, was also not a problem. In time, the sophisticated clinical practice we at Columbia so carefully developed and passionately advocated might slowly evolve in DNP programs until higher levels of commonalities in direct care would be reached. But for now, new clinical standards were considered premature. These issues were at the heart of our efforts at Columbia and CACC as we pursued certification planning. If the degree was being established without clinical standards, then certification became all the more critically important to distinguish the clinical experts among all DNP graduates. The thinking that eventually, slowly, over time, these distinctions would find their way into clinical DNP programs may be an accurate forecast. Even so, we already had a fix on new standards and wanted to institutionalize them as a goal for completing that evolution.

We also didn't find comfort in waiting for nursing to catch up and adopt standards we believed could alter the face of primary care. The shortage was worsening, with plans to place rare primary care physicians increasingly in charge of NPs, to make sure that all patients had at least nominal access to a physician. This spelled death to independent practice in nursing. We believed it was imperative for us to grab the reins of this evolving policy and to place nurses—highly qualified nurses—in charge. The medical home would work best if nurses ran these teams. Physician specialists have important roles in coordinated primary care services, but the generalist, the one who gives sophisticated care and coordinates the rest, is a role designed for a DNP clinical expert. There is a physician specialist shortage looming as well; we need to advocate the increase of these specialists while advancing our own comprehensive care. We simply weren't ready to join the crowd and play the waiting game. The urgency to establish doctoral programs for nurse administrators was, to us, far less important for the profession and patients than training and identifying the new level of nurse clinicians. Importantly, Don Melnick and his colleagues at NBME agreed with us.

CACC met in Istanbul in the spring of 2007. We had been working all year on a proposal for a specific certification exam, and it had been exciting and heady work. We emphasized to our colleagues that by taking essentially

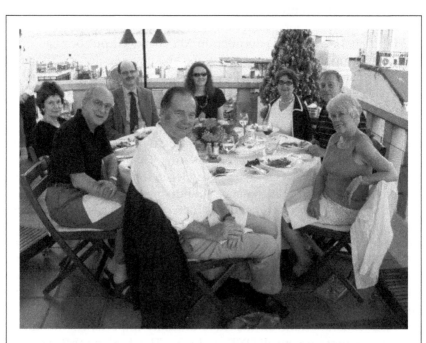

CACC group around the dinner table in Istanbul (2007). Counterclockwise beginning center front, Tom Kean, Mary Mundinger, Paul Mundinger, Ada Sue Hinshaw, Kristine Warbasse, Jerry Kleiner, Barry Cooper, and Buz Cooper.

● ● ● ● ●

the same exam as MDs, DNPs would more likely be viewed as comparable by the public—a huge benefit for us. NBME cycles questions out of the current pool used for the final step 3 of the MD licensing exam. Questions are removed from that pool if they become overused or stale. For our DNP exam, we would have an exam developed from that separate pool. Any questions deemed inaccurate or out of date would not be in the pool of questions used for our exam; only tested and reliable questions not currently in use for the MD exam would be available to us. The CACC decision in 2007 focused on exam development.

Essentially, our exam would mirror categories, numbers, and degree of difficulty in the exam for DNPs. The statisticians and other content experts at NBME would ensure that our exam would test the same competencies using the same methods and format as the MD exam. We were ecstatic that they would publicly attest to this level of comparability in the exam they were developing for our DNPs. We were also scared to death. What if the exam results showed a measurable nursing deficit? What if too many bright but unqualified DNPs took the exam and our overall results suffered? After all, MDs all get the same training, often geared to the exam. How would DNPs fare in this regard, with variable training, completed before such an exam was even contemplated? Was there a match? And what about our bravado about the Columbia model? What if it wasn't up to these standards after all? The randomized controlled trial results had given us great confidence, but this was different—it was a detailed exam covering broad and comprehensive patient care.

With great fanfare we presented the plan to CACC in the Istanbul meeting, and it was received with a cautious welcome. More and more the council approved a wide berth for these sophisticated plans, but none of the other

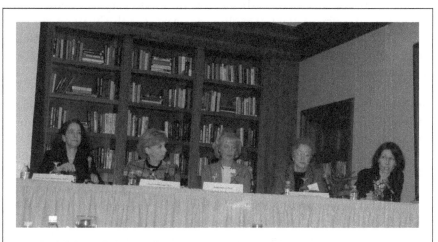

CACC (2007). From left, Judy Honig, Donna Hathaway, Joan Shaver, Patricia Starck, and Jan Smolowitz.

● ● ● ● ●

CACC nursing schools were planning to recommend the exam to their new DNP students or graduates. They didn't resist the development of such a plan; they just weren't ready for it on their own campuses. Once again the Columbia cohort was going to be in the lead, agreeing to take this highly public first exam.

In January 2009, CACC was scheduled to meet in a particularly festive celebration on a boat touring the Galapagos. We had planned the trip to mark 10 years of CACC challenges and success. Each year as CACC concluded its annual meeting we announced where the next meeting would be. In January 2008 we told everyone to save the week a year hence for the landmark 10-year anniversary. As 2008 went forward and we reached a firm date for the first DNP certification exam, we found we were on a collision course of receiving test results the day before everyone left for Ecuador. We didn't know if we would be celebrating a successful outcome or examining the failure of our daunting experiment. Even more excruciating was not having any more data than raw numbers of who passed or who failed. Several of the candidates would be on the boat, not knowing their fate.

We were deeply relieved to get the remarkable results of the exam. Half had passed, using the same passing scores of MD test takers. We had proven it was possible for nurses, with targeted education and experience, to meet the same standard in general medical care as physicians. MD equivalency wasn't our goal, but rather, comparability in the skills and knowledge needed to provide the full scope of care that patients needed and sought and that insurers would pay for. Comparability in general medical care was essential, but our more nuanced and future goal would be showing that these certified DNPs also brought extraordinarily valuable—and unique—nursing skills and approaches to their practice and to their patients. They weren't simply capable of generalist medicine. It is the DNPs exquisite combination that results in a new patient care clinician. And it is this new practitioner, with these expanded and necessary skills, who will develop and establish comprehensive care and replace the more limited primary care that has been in such deficit and disarray.

The extended Galapagos cruise allowed us to celebrate and to fully discuss what this meant to our future endeavors. Not surprisingly, the same old issues arose; resources rather than the validity of this new educational pathway were the biggest barrier. Our nurse members wanted the DNP movement to be free to experiment and diversify in order to take advantage, school by school, of the resources available, including university support. One CACC member noted that the only questions the trustees at her university had posed regarding her proposed DNP program were whether the graduates would be addressed as "doctor" and whether they would want a key to the physicians' lunch room. Other nursing schools' DNP proposals couldn't get past medical school resistance unless the DNP degree was more conventional, in practice scholarship, for example, which would appear more like a research degree program. Even those nursing deans who aspired to a clinical DNP found their faculties resistant, believing such a degree would be a second-level PhD program or in a field of scholarship not worthy of a doctoral degree. Others, who saw the potential of an equally high-level doctorate in clinical care, questioned where the clinical experts could be found who could teach and guide clinical DNP students. And those who looked very closely at DNP education saw that it would take a much higher level of faculty involvement in clinical care than conventional advanced practice programs required at the master's-degree level, where many such mentors were available.

We made progress in our 2009 meeting mostly because half of the first exam takers had passed. Progress was advanced on the recidivist issues still unresolved because it was now clear that clinical DNPs were achieving a measurable new standard of care that changed the dynamics of the meeting from how to measure this new level of care to how to break down the barriers preventing wide adoption. It was not going to be easy, but it was inevitable.

STRIVING TO INCREASE THE NUMBER OF CLINICAL DNP PROGRAMS

We at Columbia wanted very much to be part of the broader DNP movement, but we also wanted to foster the identity of clinical DNPs. Without the secure distinction, recognition would revert to the lowest common denominator. The new certification was a huge step toward establishing the distinction we sought. We at Columbia and CACC were determined to find ways to increase the number of clinical DNP programs. We believed the best and quickest way to do so was to pursue higher reimbursement for these practitioners. If certifications added to one's income, we had an incontrovertible argument for those contemplating which DNP program to enroll in.

At the same time, we wanted our brand of DNP to be part of the rapidly developing AACN standards. If we did not, we risked being outliers without the support of nursing organizations. If we were in the circle, we could continue to move clinical standards to broader adoption, and incrementally move DNP programs in our direction. It was crucial to stay within the broader national movement.

We believed that our new certification had to be nationally accredited. Currently accredited certifications in advanced practice were the key to licensure as an advanced practice nurse (APN). We wanted our certification to be accredited so that we could then act to have the exam lead to *licensure at the new level of practice*. This idea came from Jan Smolowitz and Judy Honig at Columbia, and with Jan's leadership, they began to develop and submit the extensive materials to the Institute for Certification Excellence.

During this time, from many sectors of medicine there was an undercurrent of anger, and even paranoia, about the new certification. A physician colleague alerted me to a broad-based, but anonymous, effort by a group of physicians to discredit the DNP and the certification. In a blog open only to MDs, a long (several hundred submissions) DNP discussion took place over several weeks between physicians representing all specialties. My physician colleague gave me his password so that I could read what was being said and what plan was being developed.

The discussion was mostly about their dismay over the increased authority of nurse practitioners, which they believe was worsened by the DNP degree and certification. One physician wrote, "It is the physician's fault that this has happened—by having mid-levels in the office. Trying to make a fast buck has in the end become the demise of our profession." Another wrote, "I say we need to work with them and find common ground. If we are involved collegially, we can help ensure both our continued success and that of the patients whose lives are in the balance. It is much harder to yell foul from the sidelines."

These measured responses were far outnumbered by those depicting something far more ominous. The overall idea was that I was the architect of this new advancement and that the establishment of CAPNA—which they viewed as the genesis of everything that followed—was a scheme supported by health insurance companies to make more money. These physicians believed my being a director on the UnitedHealthcare board was why the DNP and certification were developed. They believed it was a serious conflict of interest for an academic developing new programs in health care to serve on the board of a public company. Thousands of physicians, of course, have been doing so for decades, but somehow this was wrong for a nurse. Many believed that UnitedHealthcare enlisted me to develop programs to undermine physician salaries. Apparently, they were not watching or listening to what CAPNA achieved—which was reimbursement equal to that given physicians, not a lesser amount. And this same equivalency was embedded in DNP development and certification; nurse practitioners already had lower reimbursements (Medicare and Medicaid most notably) and, in our plan, the DNP movement would erase those disparities. This did not influence the bloggers' thinking, however. One physician wrote that I was "possibly implicated in various schemes, and probably stand to benefit almost directly from such an increase in DNP numbers and scope of practice." Another wrote that I was "supported by UnitedHealthcare to create a nurse practice clinic."

Actually, the CAPNA practice was established before I was appointed to the UnitedHealthcare board, and the board never gave financial support to our endeavors. Nonetheless, these bloggers pursued the evil scheme hypothesis and traced ideas on how to destroy the DNP and certification. They considered asking the Institute of Medicine to take away my membership (the conflict of interest theory) and to lobby NMBE to disband their partnership with CACC based on these same issues. They agreed whatever they decided to do should be anonymous.

And that's just what they did. They wrote a long letter of protest to NMBE president Don Melnick. There were no identifying authors of the letter and no return address. The letter was simply signed "1,041 physicians." We had always been fortunate to have physician support for our work—importantly those at Columbia, but many many others as well. And importantly, they lent their names, reputations, and honor to our work. We knew we were in the right place in terms of the medical profession, but the attack and comments from this very angry cabal were unnerving. One likes to think that physicians are above anonymous personal attacks and that personal integrity was a professional requisite. If there really were 1,041 physicians who read and agreed to the letter, why were they not willing to be identified and accountable for their claims?

MD students are taught with the NBME exams as a blueprint for their learning. DNP students, however, had no such blueprint utilized in their education. We offered an exam that tested what generalist physicians knew, and we made a leap of faith that DNP training had given the candidates knowledge to pass the exam. We believed we had chosen the correct standard, but we were a long way from assuring adequate preparation for the new test. In time that gap would narrow significantly, and those familiar with the test content and format requirements (many of whom chose to take one of the MD prep courses for licensure) would do exceedingly well on the exam. Even with these improvements, the highest scores continue to be for those who were initially NPs in adult or family practice. Interestingly, in the next 3 years of exams, the overall exam cohort had far less experience in practice as an advanced practice nurse. We may have captured (in the first exams) those who had been waiting a long time for a clinical doctorate and brought a wealth of experiential wisdom with them to the exam.

The challenge for DNP programs—especially those that are replacing MS-level advanced practice programs—is to ensure that basic and advanced diagnostic and treatment capabilities are strongly woven into DNP training. While experience counts in every trade and every profession, if we have a new level of care in nursing we must make sure that all graduates meet that challenge—and this means developing curricular and outcomes standards.

As we devoted our energies to these efforts, we knew full well that the key to the expansion of clinical DNP programs like ours was to be able to produce a sufficient number of DNPs—with certification—to provide the new faculty positions necessary to establish the programs. It would take this cohort development to fuel the expansion of the new standard of care.

In addition to providing a pool of questions that covered the new DNP competencies and holding a respected reputation for integrity in testing, we believed the NBME partnership was valuable for DNPs to be seen as comparable with MDs in basic medicine. If we had found another organization with the pool of questions we needed, there would have been no way to tie this new standard to the existing one—Medicine. The NBME partnership guaranteed the power of this comparability.

CACC CONTINUES TO STRUGGLE WITH DNP
COMPREHENSIVE CARE COMPETENCIES

CACC met next in 2010 in Capetown, South Africa. The group, with all its different priorities and challenges, shared strong bonds. Support for the clinical DNP and the certification we chose were unanimous. We knew we would always have special memories of this uncharted pathway— goal apparent but detours unexpected and unseen. It was a thrilling time. During the Capetown meeting we found ourselves discussing the same issues—how to distinguish clinical DNPs, how to use certification as a way to secure equal reimbursement, and how to assist schools to launch such programs.

In many ways we felt like actors in a Woody Allen film where no one could see the easy answer to the primary care deficit—it was nurses not physicians, and in particular the new DNP nurse. Mostly the public perception of the primary care deficit and the role of nurse practitioners looked something like this: increase the utilization of nurse practitioners, but keep them "supervised" by the few primary care physicians through the development of "medical homes." Patients would supposedly give up direct access to specialists and enroll instead in a medical home where physicians, nurse practitioners, and other professionals would provide care determined by the physician. Medical home sounds comfy and secure, but patients didn't like that system when it was called a health maintenance organization (HMO) in the 1970s and don't like it now. They like having direct access to specialists. They like looking up their symptoms or diseases on the Internet and choosing which clinician they want advice and care from. Furthermore, they don't like the constraints of office-based generalist care.

Comprehensive care practiced by DNPs is not limited to a single generalist setting. Most DNPs, in fact, provide their comprehensive care in partnership with physician specialists. Just as patients are drawn to direct access to specialists, they realize—and seek—comprehensive care as part of the package. Primary care as it was practiced in the past is a disappearing specialty. Physicians don't want to practice in that pattern, even if they are given a posse of "midlevels" whom they oversee and who actually deliver the care. Physician oversight—as well as the outdated perspective on primary care—has made this model too constrained and unattractive to patients. But comprehensive care has great promise. Even as patients select their retinue of specialists, they will have a clinician to care for them—or coordinate their care—in every setting where they receive care. DNPs as comprehensive care clinicians also focus on chronic illness care, which often is based on a disease or illness, which is the DNPs' specialty. For example, primary care tends to comprise initial contact and ongoing office-based generalist care across the spectrum of illnesses. Comprehensive care tends to be initial contact and ongoing care *and on-site engagement wherever the patient receives care.* This doesn't mean a DNP is velcroed onto a patient during his health care journey, but it does mean the DNP is on call for all those encounters. The emerging practice choice of DNPs is more often giving generalist care and oversight to patients whose majority of care is within a specialty—cardiac, cancer, neurological. These new "teams" are specialist MD plus DNP rather than generalist MD overseeing generalist NP. The content and authority and relationships are profoundly different. Even where DNPs choose an undifferentiated generalist practice, the scope of care is broader and involves more authority across sites or care than conventional primary care. DNPs are the nexus of this new movement, and they are doing so without any visionary plan in place. They are just following where their new expertise is leading them.

The year 2010 was a pivotal one for health care with the passage of the Affordable Care Act (ACA). Franklin Delano Roosevelt had secured a social safety net nearly 80 years before, and President Johnson, the wizard of Congress and newly empowered president following Kennedy's tragic death, brought guaranteed health care to the poor and elderly with the passage of Medicaid and Medicare 45 years ago. Neither of these bigger than life leaders, nor Truman who also contemplated the idea, believed they could do the same for middle-aged middle-income Americans. Now, in the face of the nation's worst financial downturn since FDR, Obama has pulled it off.

The core of the complex legislation is mandatory coverage—everyone will be required to have health insurance by 2014. The federal government would subsidize this radical transformation in several ways, including paying the states' share of the newly covered 16 million Medicaid enrollees for 3 years, and all but 10% of those added beneficiaries in years afterward. Government would also provide premium support to individuals using newly established insurance markets. Other subsidies and cross payments would also come into play. What most Americans may not have understood is that they already pay for the care of the uninsured; the new law would change the system of how patients receive care. Instead of relying on unpaid ER care or charity (public money in both cases), the newly insured would receive earlier care in more appropriate sites of care and have lifesaving chronic illness care rarely provided in ER encounters.

For us in the DNP world, we saw enormous opportunity for our new model of care in the environment and system that ACA projected. Never had nurses—and especially DNPs—been more needed.

18
•••••

Searching for Balance

•••••

In the midst of the heady advances in Doctor of Nursing Practice (DNP) certification, the nursing school was flourishing. In 2006 we had a budget of $23 million. Research revenues totaled $3.8 million, or 16.5% of all revenues. Faculty practice revenues totaled $556,000 or 2.5% of all revenues. After expenses, we had a $5 million surplus—or over 20% of our revenues—which we transferred to our endowment. The year 2006 was still a very productive year in the market, and our endowment value soared.

Our researchers were making a mark nationally. Sue Bakken, in medical informatics, Joyce Anastasi in HIV/AIDS, particularly in the area of ameliorating the devastating side effects of treatment, Kris Gebbie in reorganizing the public health workforce, Mary Byrne in the care of compromised infants and children, Dick Garfield in measuring the civilian burden of international conflict and war, Elaine Larson in infection control, and Pat Stone in the economics of health care—all were leading national figures in their areas of expertise. Several were covering their full salaries—and significant student support—from their grants, and still contributing to teaching and policy development.

Everything was coming into balance. Our faculty practice program was maturing, the practitioners were seasoned in negotiating substantive practices that fit with their academic work, and they were building the scholarly contributions to evidence the academic nature of their work. Case studies, evidence-based evaluations of their interventions, and collaborative manuscripts with members of other disciplines were increasingly showcasing their sophisticated clinical work. Researchers were following a more conventional route of external funding and publications in peer-reviewed journals. But "conventional" doesn't tell half the story of the place they were establishing for themselves. First, they were developing a research program in the school that had never before had a research presence. They were not only the entrepreneurs, but they were being so without any layer of senior grounded research faculty to support them. And the niche each of them established was unique and not a graft onto existing work elsewhere. They were groundbreaking, and they did it without any "conventional environment." Most interesting is that all of the research studies transcended traditional nursing research. Reading the studies and the meaning of the studies, one would see that the findings enriched nursing, but they did more: These scholars touched on the broader health care field and focused on economics, ethics, and policy. They were clearly members of a broad research community, publishing in journals where nurses were rarely the authors.

Research and practice were two distinguishing parts of the school, but educational initiatives filled our portfolios as well. As areas of practice or policy developed nationally—and internationally—our faculty were among the first to develop curricula and student experiences to cover newly identified competencies; genetics, ethics, health policy, practice management, informatics, biostatistics all expanded in Columbia nursing programs in these years.

In 2007, research revenues reached a new high. With only 12 research faculty, research revenues reached an annual high of $4.5 million. It was a remarkable achievement. We began building a program of financial support for doctoral students. The outstanding funding success of researchers provided the majority of funds for this advancement, but we also had the now-recurring multimillion dollar surplus each year, allowing investments in doctoral education as well as our endowment growth.

By 2007 we had endowed 11 chairs and five faculty were tenured. We felt we were beginning to anchor a secure future for the school. The one annoyance that kept showing up was the disparity in common costs that we paid. In a zero-sum game it was hard to argue our "need," but the facts were that we were charged 36% of revenues, Dental was charged 20% of theirs, and Public Health 12% (one fourth of ours!) The only way out was to develop "need," and a new building would solve that—and a lot more.

Interest in the DNP program was growing and alumni support was strong. The original alumni association kept their firewall in place, making sure their identity did not disappear, but that identity was more and more outdated and frail. It was a cultural dissonance more than a professional one, and it continued to be a dividing line between the old and new school.

In 2008, the faculty was deeply engaged in revamping the two doctoral programs (research and practice) so that each mirrored the other in equal—but different—ways to achieve a high level of scholarship. The way was to require full-time study and provide full tuition support. We did this when we transitioned the Doctor of Nursing Science (DNSc) to PhD in 2008, but full-time study was not an attractive choice for most Doctor of Nurse Practitioner (DNP) applicants. Early in the history of DNP education most students were seasoned advanced practice nurses with good jobs and salaries. They did not want to resign those positions to become full-time DNP students.

Doctoral tuition support came with an expectation of significant engagement in their program of study, learning the scholarship aspects, independent practice, or independent research. The DNP students would have incurred a significant financial shortfall, whereas most PhD students had not developed a similar level of salary or authority. As the DNP program matured, and Columbia students in the Entry to Practice (ETP) program increasingly aspired for DNP enrollments, a full-time DNP program became possible; ETP students are all full time, so it was an easier transition to full-time DNP study than for those leaving a high-paid practice in order to enroll.

In 2008, our NIH ranking moved from 27 to 13. We were particularly gratified to once again have our research faculty cohort number one in per capita funding.

We had begun a fund (separate from endowment deposits) to fund a new building. In 2008, we had $18 million in the fund (cash and pledges) toward a $30 million down payment for the building. We expected to have the $30 million within 3 years, which Vice President Lee Goldman had asked us to do in order for him to approve us to "reestablish" our building campaign. We submitted a plan on September 3, 2008 to fund a $160 million building with $25 million from the university, $25 million from our endowment, and $110 million in debt. If our proportionate growth continued (including increased costs of debt and running a large building), we believed the costs could be met and the endowment replenished to $100 million in 8 years. Our endowment was held partly in the university and partly in the Columbia Presbyterian funds. We kept getting richer but no closer to Goldman's approval for a new building; even this new plan was met with silence.

The medical center began a process of reconfiguring the finances of each school in order to build a central reserve, which would be used for expenditures that would benefit the common good. Those of us not in the medical school weren't sure this was a good thing; the vice president who decided expenditures was also dean of the medical school—at best he'd have two votes to each of our one vote, and we weren't even sure how the list of possible expenditures would be developed or evaluated.

Adding to our wariness was the 10% tax to be charged on *increased* tuition revenues; nursing and public health were the only schools projecting such increases. In this reconfiguration, there would not only be reassessment of medical center shared costs, but also a reconfiguration of how common costs to the central university would be split between the health sciences schools. In the "old" configuration, nursing was (in my opinion) overcharged: in terms of common costs as a percent of *expenditures* in the current assessment:

Medicine	19%
Public Health	9%
Dentistry	21%
Nursing	26%

In the new configuration, nursing would take on new "common" debt. The outcome of common costs as a percent of expenditures:

Medicine	17%	down 2% from current
Public Health	12%	up 3% from current
Dentistry	29%	up 8% from current
Nursing	40%	up 14% from current

I was dismayed and shared the plan with faculty at a meeting on April 28, 2009, and met with Goldman to protest the inequities. Not only did nothing change, but in a June 16, 2008 letter to me regarding approval of nursing's 2009 budget, he stated: "As you know, our collective future is critically dependent on solid financial performance that builds operating surpluses for investments in education, research and clinical initiatives." This statement is exactly what we in nursing had been doing for years; we just had questions about the "collective" nature of the new plan.

As I wrote the narrative for the budget submission to Goldman on March 6, 2008, I noted that our endowment had reached $100 million. We had done so through productivity and thrift. We were not eager to financially support the medical school, but the new financial arrangements contributed to that subsidy. This (and the undue delay on our building) were leading to growing contention between the nursing school and medical administration, and between the School of Public Health and the administration. Dentistry was in a somewhat different situation since they shared a building and 2 years of classes with the medical school. The consolidation of finances and debt resulted in a loss of shared purpose and individual accountability. Things were fraying.

In 2010 the Affordable Care Act was passed, presaging an unbelievable opportunity for advanced practice nursing. Where else would the nation's newly enfranchised 32 million individuals find primary care? The 4-year phase-in period presented us with new energy to accomplish the next steps for DNPs—national recognition of our certification and then approval to have our certification count for licensure at this new higher level of practice. And we would need to make the case with insurers to pay us as they do primary care physicians so that the new beneficiaries would have access to nurse practitioners on a par with physician practitioners. We had a lot to accomplish, but the path was clear, very clear.

Research was thriving as well. We had 23 active grants with total multiyear values of $22.7 million. Our 2010 budget projected total revenues of $28 million, with the new central tax applied for the first time: Our share would be $5,791,000, or more than 20% of our revenues. The detailed list of support to be provided included wet and dry lab space and animal care support (of which we had none), sponsored project support and campus housing subsidy (of which we had a small part of expenses), a general operating assessment for the vice president/dean of medicine offices and a new common cost assessment that would be shared equally by the four schools.

Early in the year I announced to the faculty that I would be leaving the dean position at the end of the year. It was time to go. My decision was made easier by the fact that my husband was combatting a fierce disease—one that would kill him in less than 2 years—and I wanted to be with him and devote myself to saving him. We added two new professorships during this transition—one named for me and one for Senator Ted Kennedy.

I planned to return after a long sabbatical and found new inspiration and hope in being named the first Edward M. Kennedy Professor in Health Policy. I had a new professional challenge as well as a personal one, and these consumed me, but there was nostalgia and sadness at leaving my place as head of the venerable and worthy school. It was part of my life and my history, and I would miss the extraordinarily bright, gifted, and kind individuals there who became my friends.

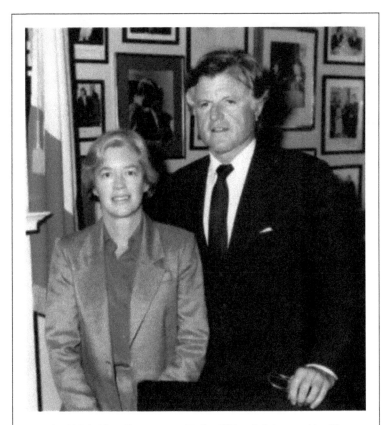

In 1984, Mundinger, as a Robert Wood Johnson Health Policy Fellow served in the Senate Labor Committee on the staff of Senator Edward Kennady.

• • • • •

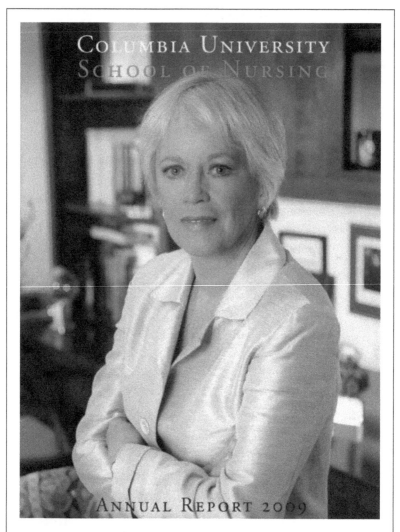

*2010 completes a quarter century as dean
(Annual Report cover, 2009).*

Section VI

•••••

Reflections:
1985–2010

•••••

ཕུལ་དུ་བྱུང་བ།

19

• • • • •

A Quarter Century of Columbia Nursing

• • • • •

DURING MY 25 YEARS AS DEAN, major accomplishments were achieved in each of the following 5-year periods, supported and often led by sustaining service from my "brain trust."

1985–1990

The years 1985–1990 marked a period of revitalizing and redefining the nursing school and its programs. It was a revolutionary and fast-paced time. We were attempting to outlast the university's inclinations to close us down, and we were fighting off Presbyterian Hospital, which wanted to reclaim us as their own. These were, in a frustrating way, competing forces that made our path forward a political as well as a financial one. Embedded in those two forces was our underlying and fundamental commitment to build the best school of nursing in the world. Unleashed from conventional ways of doing things because of the severity of our situation, we could be innovative and make decisions quickly. We were free to develop research and practice in our own self-defined, and often unique, ways. And we changed our educational programs radically as well. Since university and hospital expectations of our success were low, our work was under the radar in terms of the chances we were taking, the wealthy and influential individuals we found to support us, and the large number of faculty and administrative recruits we could hire, who joined to make changes, not to anchor the past. It all worked out, but certainly not as the early skeptics had projected. Our major accomplishment in this first 5-year period was the establishment of faculty practice.

1990–1995

During 1990–1995 we developed the first nursing doctorate in health services research in the country, which had the added value of capturing the

195

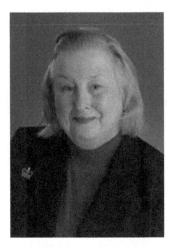

*Sarah Cook, vice dean,
Brain Trust at Columbia*

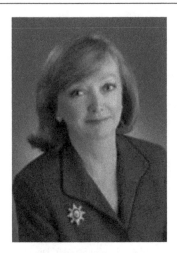

*Jennifer Smith, senior
associate dean for
Development, Brain
Trust at Columbia*

● ● ● ● ●

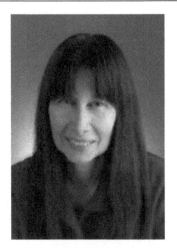

*Jan Smolowitz, senior
associate dean
for Practice, Brain
Trust at Columbia*

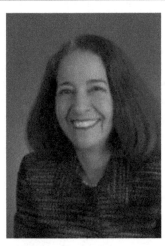

*Judy Honig, associate dean
for Student Services, Brain
Trust at Columbia*

● ● ● ● ●

● ● ● ● ●

outcomes of our practice initiatives. We began to make significant inroads in recruiting research faculty, and receiving our first National Institutes of Health (NIH) awards, beginning with a brilliant scholar, practitioner, and researcher, Joyce Anastasi.

In this period we also established our first landmark practice, when we opened an independent nurse practitioner (NP) primary care practice and conducted the first randomized controlled trial (RCT) comparing NP and MD practices. Dr. William Speck, president of Presbyterian Hospital, Dr. Mike Weisfeldt, chair of Medicine, and Dr. Herb Pardes, vice president of Health Services, paved the way for this multitiered effort, a first for the hospital to recognize the nursing school faculty practice model.

During this period, the school celebrated its Centennial, something very few would have expected in the dark days of 1985. As a mark of our financial success and conservatism, we ended the year with a surplus equal to the money we spent, and we transferred it to our rapidly growing endowment.

1995–2000

The 5-year period from 1995 until 2000 was primarily devoted to expanding and grounding our enterprise, establishing endowed chairs, and opening Columbia Advanced Practice Nurse Associates (CAPNA). The RCT results were in, were entirely positive, and published in the *Journal of the American Medical Association (JAMA)* with great fanfare. We rattled the medical world with our ability to secure par reimbursement from insurance companies for care of commercially insured patients, and *60 Minutes* with Morley Safer, celebrated our achievements. The new accelerated BS program for college graduates was flooded with applicants, many because they wanted to walk in the path of Columbia' Center for Advanced Practice (CAP) and CAPNA pioneers. Our finances were exceedingly strong. Our new international council to help advocate for our new model of care was active and thriving.

2000–2005

From 2000 to 2005 our researchers' record in NIH awards reached first place in the nation in the percentage of research faculty who were funded by NIH. No school did better than ours. We established our new practice model as the DNP degree, and we worked ceaselessly to develop standards for the degree. We graduated the first DNP students in early 2005. We recognized that national clinical standards that reached the level of our graduates would take many years to accomplish; the new degree was wildly popular across the profession, but standards were so variable as to be uncodifiable.

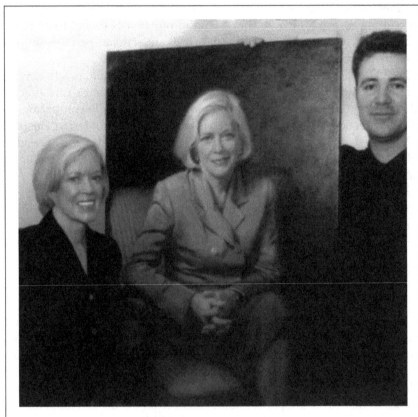

Paul Newton, portraitist (2004).

• • • • •

2005–2010

From 2005 until 2010, while keeping our goal of establishing high clinical standards for the DNP, we changed our strategy from *degree* standards to those reached through certifications. Developing a partnership with the National Board of Medical Examiners (NBME) was a crowning achievement because of NBME's stellar reputation in testing and because the nursing exam would be composed of reliable questions that covered our new practice. The added benefit, showing the medical comparability with MD test takers, would add public credibility. Dr. Don Melnick, head of the NBME, one of our heroes, made this possible.

During these 25 years a new building to house our increasingly exceptional faculty and their work was elusive. Convincing our nursing colleagues that a strong and identifiable clinical doctorate would be the best outcome for this new degree was not possible during these first few years. We celebrated

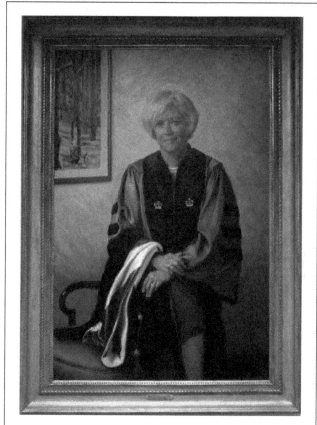

*Paul Newton paints a new rendition of
the dean (2010).*

● ● ● ● ●

the fact that a new degree—the first doctoral degree in practice—had been possible and that we were in the forefront. In time, as resources (and understanding of the new role) grow, the clinical DNP will become the standard. And a new building is already on the horizon as I write this. Those long sequestered funds would finally be invested in an edifice worthy of our endeavors.

The 25 years of my deanship were enabled and fostered by courageous, brilliant, and enormously talented faculty. We shared an emerging vision as it played out on the national stage, and a quarter of a century went by in a flash of excitement, trepidation, celebration, and enduring friendship.

20
•••••

Personal Advice to the Reader
•••••

A NEW CHAPTER IN MY PROFESSIONAL life is opening up for me as I close the one I began 25 years ago. As the Edward M. Kennedy Professor, I return to my health policy roots. With the imprimatur of this great man, I have a head start in making a difference in America's struggle to provide everyone with guaranteed health care. Using nursing as an instrument of this mission, I believe all we did at Columbia will support my new pathway. Because my direction is away from administration, I can look at those past achievements in a fresh light, undimmed by any conflicting efforts to remain in an administrative role. I know what helped me succeed, and there are rules, advice, and perspective that may be useful. I can provide some ideas to those who are embarking on leadership and administrative positions.

First, the two are profoundly different. *Leadership* means sticking your neck out ahead of those whom you hope will follow, and *administration* is managing and guiding those who may or may not want to take a new pathway. Combining the two has inherent conflicts but provides a system for change. It is a careful ballet. Administration is built on a conservative base, whereas leadership is radical. There are many ways to manage this duality, and I will share with you what some of those strategies are.

First, it is difficult indeed to be a leader if you don't have potential followers. If you have a mission, or even a strategy to change a short-term situation, you need standing where you can exert your viewpoint. It could be an administrative position, but in academia that is a big challenge. Academia is, almost by definition, a conservative bastion of limited change; new ideas thrive in this environment, but actions to operationalize ideas happen elsewhere. If you are a dean interested in change, you will almost always find the power to make change come from the private sector. You can do one of two things: raise money for your school from those who support your change agenda, or secure positions of influence within organizations

201

external to your university where their views will add credibility to yours. Here are two examples:

1. When I needed desperately to increase nursing's presence in the university, I chose to develop a group of advisors whom the university already knew and revered.
2. When I needed to get professional acceptance from colleagues for our new ideas at Columbia, I sought support from organizations that nursing revered.

These were different constituencies for different reasons. High-profile business leaders advocating for my ideas helped with university support; high-profile health care organizations that financially supported our ideas were influential in nursing. You need both. But how do you accomplish this? Always—always—focus your pitch on what is in it for the advocate you are pitching, not what's in it for you. For those of eminence in the private sector, build the case that your project has potential to be standard setting and will burnish their own reputations as visionaries. For foundations or other funding agencies, make it clear that their support will set them apart—and ahead as recognizing important trends. Universities care about their reputations, and support for your agenda from recognized leaders or visionaries will influence university support for your ideas. Funding of course is important in its own right—dollars have influence—but those dollars are worth more when they are from a prestigious source. Everyone wants to feel their support for an untested idea has lots of company from individuals and organizations they respect. It's all about reputation, self-interest, and self-advancement. Choose your supporters with care. Be elitist.

Second, present your ideas for change to faculty in the same vein. Make sure the changes you want will add value to those who must bring about the change. Support them in the ways that will prevent pushback or rebellion. Give them performance and financial rewards for signing on to the change process. Titles are free but persuasive; give advantageous titles to those who follow your lead. Give bonuses where their support adds financial gain to your school. Make change an institutional advancement, not your personal one. Craft changes—honestly—in how they will benefit the faculty and your organization. Make your vision their vision.

Surprisingly, this is not a difficult way to lead. After all, being a successful leader means leading a successful organization. It's all derivative. If your organization or faculty succeeds, so do you. Unfortunately, many deans see themselves caught in the tide of faculty opinion. Wherever the water ebbs and flows, they want to stay afloat. This is a terrible dynamic, leading too often to a defeating standstill when progress could be attained. After all, a tide is meant to bring in new life, and it can be a source of change. One only has to grasp those opportunities. Faculty, as all of us, are wary of change that requires new ways of thinking and doing, but if we can see where change can benefit us, it makes all the difference in how we respond. Leaders must show their constituents how they specifically will profit from the efforts it will take to change the status quo.

This isn't a duplicitous strategy. Why would any dean (or leader in another venue) advocate change that would be deleterious to its membership? The success is in the ability to link those benefits to the current efforts of those whom you need to bring about change. This challenge requires a leader with strong and honest beliefs, and the charisma to enlist the support of those crucial to success. And it takes courage so that you can bridge that gap. If you don't have that kind of strong belief and personal courage, you should pursue a different career.

The most tragic and personally diminishing path a leader can take is when she (or he) perceives the ultimate—and best—outcome, but lacks the courage or will to reach toward that vision. Settling for a lesser goal—unless it is a clear next step toward a loftier one—is a waste of leadership potential. Worse, it can lead to a road to mediocrity for the enterprise the individual has been chosen to lead, saps resources and support for future endeavors, and through such passivity gives strength to forces that are not in the best interest of the "leader's" constituency. This neglect, born of the choice to take the easy road, where support is readily available from the conservative majority, is the villainy of poor leadership. Those leaders who coast toward the seemingly safe shallows are doomed to a rocky finish. "Leaders" who act this way are not leaders, but are instead attempting to secure their current position rather than their lasting legacy.

In terms of enlisting political and financial support, you will need an inner core group of individuals with whom you can share mission and strategy and tactics. They must feel this is their mission along with yours. In order to do this you must—must—personally believe in your mission. Authenticity is powerful. You cannot sell a system or product you don't' fully believe in. If it is someone else's mission—that of your organization or your university—but not yours, you will fail. Real change occurs when leaders are infused with the belief that such change is fundamentally needed. If you cannot get really involved in the outcome, don't expect others to do so. It's all up to you. The alternative is to go with the flow; accommodate your faculty or your university and hold the reins without offering direction. This is not leadership, although it may be a weak system of administration.

My own experience and belief is that those who bring about change work on a time frame that is fundamentally different from those who don't envision the same clear outcome. Incrementalism has its value, but only if used strategically toward a bold new goal. I have learned that pushing beyond expected conservative time frames is crucial to success. In 1985 when Presbyterian Hospital wanted to "save" Columbia nursing by adopting it as a stepchild (or renegade child coming back after years of profligate excess), this was not a time for collaboration. If we had not escaped by flagrant exceptionalism, we would have been consumed by the better grounded conservative hospital enterprise. This would have been lethal for our school.

It's easy to say "build an external constituency and raise money," but these are goals worth your every effort. We saved as much money as we did because we were unable to spend to build a new building. Had we been given that approval I am certain we would have more quickly advanced our research presence, which I fervently wish we could have done. But this would have reduced the recognition we were achieving by building such an unprecedented endowment. With our practice initiatives extending into space we didn't pay for (the 30 plus faculty practices on the medical center), we didn't need space for our clinical endeavors. But the power of our huge endowment reduced university opposition to our many radical initiatives. Money is power. I cannot underestimate the importance of raising money. In a cramped financial situation, spend preferentially on good fundraising. This is far easier in a private institution than in a public one. However, my observations are that leaders of public institutions are too quick to default to their received limitations in raising money. I don't think the acceptance of public funding necessarily neuters one's ability to get additional private funding; the National Institutes of Health and foundation grants attest to the potential. The view that publicly funded entities depend on public funding as the sole source of revenue is suicidal. Entrepreneurial activities can thrive in any environment. Push the boundaries. I don't know of any organization or university that asks that private funds be returned.

What if you are not in New York City but want to develop major business support for your enterprise? What if you are in the Midwest, far from the nation's business elite? You don't have to look far. Look to your own regional business leaders, who hold sway with your organization or university, or look to regional offices of leading national organizations. Find alumni from your university (not just your school) who might have a stake in health care. Find out who from your region or university sits on corporate boards or executive positions in industries related to health care. Meet with them. Tell them about your riveting new ideas. Solicit their advice, not their dollars; that will come later.

Review the membership of the health/finance committees in the U.S. Senate and Congress and in your state congressional offices. Meet with those in the U.S. Congress from your state on the health and finance committees. Meet with staff and executives at Health and Human Services that oversee the major governmental programs in health care—Medicare, Medicaid, and the Veterans Administration. Find ways to make your agenda their agenda.

Just as titles are free, so are awards. Have your organization or school give annual expansively named awards to those who can further your agenda. Everyone likes having a piece of crystal or a framed certificate on their bookshelf attesting to their eminence. Design beautiful and attractive awards and titles to be given to those who are in positions of influence to foster your mission. And call on them afterward to keep helping you.

All of these approaches are targeted to make your agenda their agenda. If you are honest and careful, it can be very influential. And basically, this brings nursing into a broader community of business and health care leaders, breaching the constraints that nursing as a profession has inadequately addressed within the small health care community.

In addition to raising the profile of your organization or school, you must do the same for yourself. There are many ways to do this, but again I would not recommend an incremental approach. Do not take lower-level board memberships or engage in association scut work. This might label you as a good citizen in your profession, but that won't get you anywhere. Stay away from any appointments that are not at a very high level. Nonprofit boards are simply a drain on your time and productivity. People like me who have already made their mark should serve on those boards. We owe it to them and have experience to be valuable. But on your own personal trajectory, aim for board membership on publicly traded companies or major foundations, which essentially function as businesses. First of all, this will be an incredible experience in how to take private company management expertise to your own initiatives. But it will also immediately place you in a different sphere of influence. Sounds good, but how do you make that happen? There are two ways.

On either tack, the first step is to identify public companies that have a connection to health care. Get a list of their executives and board members. Do some research on these individuals and see where they live and where they went to college, and if they have credentials as professionals in health care.

Prioritize these companies so that you have a list of those who are most impacted by nurses, advanced practice nurses in particular. Which companies care about nurses prescribing medications? Home care? Devices that patients have to learn and be supervised to use? Informatics? (Nurses have always been more enthusiastic than other health professionals in adopting communication advances.) Also consider nutrition supplement organizations, national chains of gym and spa organizations, makers of assistive devices, commercial insurers. Look more closely to see where their corporate offices are and whether any are in your region. You will find several potential matches with your institution, your profession, and your own background.

Second, look at your own institution's leadership (executives, trustees) to see if any have connections to your list of preferred companies. Have they been involved with any of those industries, or might they be alumni from the same college as some of the CEOs or board members?

Third, take a look at any corporate or business funding your school or institution has received. Is there a potential advocate there who could introduce you or send your name to a related company as a potential board member?

Once you have a list of CEOs/trustees of a company to whom you could offer advice, think carefully how you would want to be introduced. While nursing will be core to your contribution, your university standing will matter, but it's not likely to be helpful to use those distinctions as your best reason to be considered for board membership. Your eminence in nursing, as someone who can advise how the profession can be useful in company plans for marketing or profit, is more riveting. You must make that connection: Your potential value is to inform a company about how to leverage nursing to further its product. But it is far more than that. If a company has a product that depends on a nurse's use or choice of that product, then you, in your eminence, become the Good Housekeeping Seal of Approval. So you will need to sell your standing in the profession, not necessarily your own personal achievements (they may be the same at times).

What this approach suggests is that you need to redesign your CV so that your eminence within your profession stands out, but also your achievements should show valued qualities public company board members may share; your executive and administrative successes, your participation in distinguished panels or research that are outside of nursing, your publications in mainstream health care journals. You need to be seen as a nurse in a broader world than nursing, but at the same time as someone who speaks for nursing in those venues.

As with any campaign, you need to get others to speak on your behalf. That's why cultivation of leaders is so critical in the earliest stages of your career. Ask for advice. Everyone appreciates being recognized as an expert. That doesn't mean all those experts will respond to your requests. To increase your chances, think—again—what you can do for those you want to be your colleagues. Authentic praise for their accomplishments is useful, but famous people aren't necessarily moved by your accolades; think of unique ways to gain their attention and support. Do you share interest in the same charity, or did they graduate from your university? It's a small world, and you can find a way once you target the person you want to become a friend of your organization. For those of you who wish someday to be a dean and gain the stage to act on your own dreams, the advice is the same. Build eminence in your own profession, but be a standout on health care. You will need those external viewpoints and support when your faculty or university makes their assessment of the potential quality of your leadership (and I do expect you want to lead, not administrate, or you wouldn't have bothered to read this book).

Know what your standards are and don't compromise them. You will never be happy in a career path that you know is less than what you believe in. That doesn't mean you shouldn't know when to compromise—and this you must do at times. Give in to others' ideas or demands when they won't fundamentally alter your ultimate goal, even though they may appear to be major concessions. In fact it's a good thing if you appear to be making major concessions; you will convince people you are a team player, which is always comforting to those you want to influence. Keep your eye on the fundamental goal you are working toward. You don't have to be Joan of Arc to show your resolve; you could be the next Margaret Thatcher instead.

You can accomplish big things if you remember the small ones. Take very good care of your staff, especially those closest to you. They know you best, and their loyalty can spell success or failure. The closer your colleagues are to your own stature, the less you need to care for them. They know they're good, and you just have to keep doing as well as they do. But staff or junior faculty can be extremely problematic for you in reaching your goals because they can sabotage you for slights you may not even know you committed.

"To thine own self be true" is profound advice, but it's a little passive. If you see an important breakthrough in social or health advancement that you could achieve—individually or as a leader—go for it. You will never regret giving your all to a worthy goal. Even if you "fail" (if you are not first over the goal line), you may change the speed in which good things happen, and that, too, is success.

Columbia School of Nursing in 2010 was very different from the school I inherited in 1985. We had developed two doctoral programs—in research and in practice—; moved all of our programs to the graduate level, including an innovative program for college graduates to study nursing; launched faculty practice; and funded research programs; all of which were new and meaningful, and were rich layers of a stronger school.

The exceptional faculty—all 100 except for one—were hired by me. Only Sarah Sheets Cook preceded my deanship, and she was my mainstay for 25 years.

Half of all alumni, over its 100-plus-year history, graduated while I was dean, and our vibrant new Alumni Association gave gravitas to our long history of eminence.

When I turned over the deanship, our endowment had topped $108 million, the highest of any school of nursing, and far more than the paltry $1 million (after paying our debts) in the dark days of 1985.

Everyone in the school contributed to these stunning achievements. It was great fun, and formed a colorful part of the fabric of our careers.

ENDOWED PROFESSORSHIPS IN RESEARCH
AND PRACTICE SCHOLARSHIP

During the years 1985–2010 the first endowed professorships were established at Columbia University School of Nursing by the Columbia University Board of Trustees. Most professorships are for outstanding researchers, but some, uniquely, are for distinguished practitioners. This was a visible recognition of the complementary and equally valuable resources developed during my tenure as dean. Four professorships honor alumni, and four honor past deans; two are in health policy, a particular interest of mine throughout my career. Two were established by friends of the school, and one in honor of Henrik Bendixen who kept the school safe while we, the faculty, made it great.

Centennial Professor in Health Policy
Anna C. Maxwell Professor in Research
Alumni Professor
Helen Pettit Professor
Herbert and Florence Irving Professor in Nursing Oncology (in their will)
Henrik Bendixen Professor in International Nursing
Professor in Pharmaceutical Therapeutics
Mary Dickey Lindsay Professor of Women's Health
Elizabeth Standish Gill Professor
Elise Fish and Stone Foundation
Dorothy M. Rogers Professor
Edward M. Kennedy Professor of Health Policy
Mary O'Neil Mundinger Professor (for each succeeding CUSON dean)

Appendix A

• • • • •

A Dean's Primer on Establishing a Clinical Doctoral Program

• • • • •

- Define the rationale and benefits for faculty to make this commitment.
- Determine the resources you will need:
  - Clinical Doctor of Nursing Practice consultants
  - Money
  - Sites
  - Medical colleagues
- Show how all faculty—researchers, educators, administrators, and clinicians—will be involved. Protect against schisms.
- Begin by identifying or recruiting faculty whose commitment is to advanced clinical practice.
- Design a faculty practice role (in conventional advanced practice) in a medical center hospital, if possible.
- Devise and put in place a faculty salary component that is acceptable to the practice site and to faculty.
- Concurrently work with top hospital executives (including nursing) and top medical school administrators (including the chair of medicine) to begin linking academic nursing resources with hospital and medical goals.
- Bring in established clinical DNP clinicians to work with you as consultants.
- Lead your faculty in developing a plan to move nursing faculty practice to a higher level. Involve everyone including the hospital head of nursing.
- Concurrently work on establishing this goal with medicine and the hospital. Detail how cross-site sophisticated care by advanced nurse practitioners can save money for the hospital (less use of resources, earlier discharge) and give physicians more time for highly specialized care.

- Enlist medical school physicians in working one on one with a small group of faculty nurse practitioners to teach them the processes of emergency room evaluation and inpatient management.
- Design courses for sophisticated clinical management with physician colleagues; pay them for their time.
- Give physicians who assist with these activities awards, honors, and opportunities to coauthor publications in non-nursing journals regarding the establishment of this new nursing practice.
- Garner external support for your new degree program by establishing a national and regional presence on an advisory board, including business and medical leaders.
- Develop relationships with state legislators who are most involved in health legislation.
- If you already have a DNP program, all you need to do is develop the clinical piece and substitute it for the original focus.
- If you don't have a DNP program, begin developing the nonclinical courses concurrently with the clinical ones.
- Develop relationships with U.S. representatives and senators from your state, particularly those on health or finance committees. Show them the quality and financial benefits of DNP practice.

Appendix B

•••••

Observations on the Laws of Leadership and Change

•••••

- Administration and leadership are not the same thing, and require different skills and approaches.
- These two roles can conflict with each other
- Leadership is standing in front of your constituency and asking others to follow.
- Administration is standing behind and pushing them forward.
- Administration requires management of the status quo.
- Leadership requires external support to give constituencies confidence in a new path.
- Leadership requires a measurable goal, promising strategy, and identifiable beneficiaries.
- Change occurs best when those whose actions are needed will be the greatest beneficiaries.
- Celebrate, with awards and honors and titles and membership, all those whose support you need.
- Give your most skeptical colleagues a seat at the table.
- Listen to those who are against your plan and use what you learn to strengthen your tactics; goals don't change, but the way to accomplish them may have to be altered. Add ammunition against would-be naysayers by showing how they could benefit by your plan.
- Never give up.
- Keep your sense of humor.
- Develop new friends and advocates and strengthen your bonds to the old ones.
- Try a new strategy.
- Keep your message and goals clear.
- Try not to wear a sign on your forehead that says, "I'm smarter then you are."
- And raise money, lots of money.

Index